World Clinics

Fungal Infections
Topical Treatments

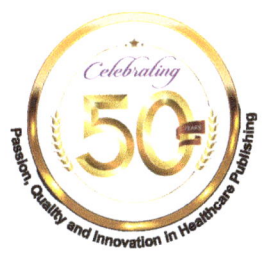

World Clinics

Dermatology

Fungal Infections
Topical Treatments

Editor-in-Chief
Rashmi Sarkar MD MNAMS

Guest Editor
Surabhi Sinha MD DNB MNAMS

2019 Volume 5 Number 1

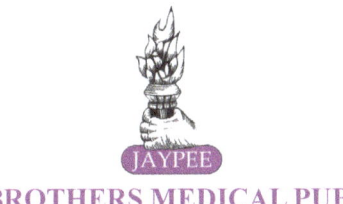

JAYPEE BROTHERS MEDICAL PUBLISHERS
The Health Sciences Publisher
New Delhi | London | Panama

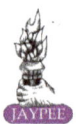 **Jaypee Brothers Medical Publishers (P) Ltd**

Headquarters

Jaypee Brothers Medical Publishers (P) Ltd
4838/24, Ansari Road, Daryaganj
New Delhi 110 002, India
Phone: +91-11-43574357
Fax: +91-11-43574314
Email: jaypee@jaypeebrothers.com

Overseas Offices

J.P. Medical Ltd
83 Victoria Street, London
SW1H 0HW (UK)
Phone: +44 20 3170 8910
Fax: +44 (0)20 3008 6180
Email: info@jpmedpub.com

Jaypee-Highlights Medical Publishers Inc
City of Knowledge, Bld. 235, 2nd Floor, Clayton
Panama City, Panama
Phone: +1 507-301-0496
Fax: +1 507-301-0499
Email: cservice@jphmedical.com

Jaypee Brothers Medical Publishers (P) Ltd
Bhotahity, Kathmandu, Nepal
Phone: +977-9741283608
Email: kathmandu@jaypeebrothers.com

Website: www.jaypeebrothers.com
Website: www.jaypeedigital.com

Cover images: (*Left*) Atypical tinea—Tinea faciei involving unilateral ear lobe. *Courtesy:* Surabhi Sinha, Sidharth Tandon, Rashmi Sarkar. (*Middle*) Onychomycosis of all fingernails. *Courtesy:* Somodyuti Chandra, Indrashis Podder. (*Right*) Tinea recidivans: New lesions of dermatophytosis occurring at the periphery of the healing lesions. *Courtesy:* Sheetanshu Kumar, Vinay Keshavamurthy.

WORLD CLINICS DERMATOLOGY: Fungal Infections Topical Treatments

2019, Volume 5, Number 1

ISSN: 2347-7156

ISBN: 978-93-5270-998-4

Printed in India

Contributors

Editor-in-Chief

Rashmi Sarkar MD MNAMS
Professor
Department of Dermatology, STD and Leprosy
Maulana Azad Medical College and Lok Nayak Hospital
New Delhi, India

Guest Editor

Surabhi Sinha MD DNB MNAMS
Consultant Dermatologist
Department of Dermatology and STD
Dr Ram Manohar Lohia Hospital and Post Graduate Institute of
Medical Education Research
New Delhi, India

Contributing Authors

Akansha Bhargava MD
Senior Resident
Department of Dermatology, Venereology and Leprosy
Bundelkhand Medical College
Sagar, Madhya Pradesh, India

Indrashis Podder MD DNB
RMO cum Clinical Tutor
Department of Dermatology
College of Medicine and Sagore Dutta Hospital
Kolkata, West Bengal, India

Isha Narang MD MRCP (SCE)
Specialist Registrar (Dermatology)
University Hospitals of Derby and Burton
United Kingdom

Mala Bhalla MD
Professor
Department of Dermatology, Venereology and Leprosy
Government Medical College and Hospital
Chandigarh, Punjab, India

Monika MD
Senior Resident
Department of Dermatology, Venereology and Leprosy
Government Medical College and Hospital
Chandigarh, Punjab, India

Neha Dubey MD
Consultant Dermatologist
Medanta The Medicity Hospital and Meraki Skin Clinic
Gurugram, Haryana, India

Nisha V Parmar MD
Specialist Dermatologist
Department of Dermatology
Rashid Hospital, Dubai Health Authority
Dubai, United Arab Emirates

Priyanka Sharma MD
Senior Resident
Department of Dermatology, Venereology and Leprosy
Government Medical College and Hospital
Chandigarh, Punjab, India

Sheetanshu Kumar MD
Senior Resident
Department of Dermatology, Venereology and Leprology
Postgraduate Institute of Medical Education and Research
Chandigarh, Punjab, India

Sidharth Tandon MD
Consultant Dermatologist
Yashoda Hospital
Ghaziabad, Uttar Pradesh, India

Sneha Ghunawat MD DNB
Consultant Dermatologist and Cosmetologist
Meraki Skin Clinic
Gurugram, Haryana, India
Fellowship ISD, Phillipines
Clinical Observership, NUH, Singapore, Fellowship IADVL (Trichology)

Somodyuti Chandra MD DNB SCE (UK)
Fellow, Venkat Center for Skin and Plastic Surgery
Bengaluru, Karnataka, India

Vinay Keshavamurthy MD DNB MRCP MNAMS
Assistant Professor
Department of Dermatology, Venereology and Leprology
Postgraduate Institute of Medical Education and Research
Chandigarh, Punjab, India

Contents

World Clin Dermatol. 2019;5(1):xi.

Editorial

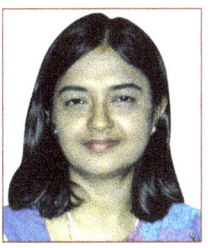

Rashmi Sarkar MD MNAMS
Editor-in-Chief

Fungal diseases are common dermatologic complaints in medical practice and definitely one of the commonest skin infections seen worldwide. Antifungal agents can be used both topically and systemically; however, systemic agents are reserved for more widespread or severe fungal infections. Dermatophytoses are usually amenable to topical agents if localized, but may need oral antifungals if multisite infection is present or the dermatophytosis is at certain areas like soles, nails, or scalp, etc.

Topical antifungals have limited but important indications. Although, the older azoles have been there for long, newer ones like luliconazole, eberconazole and sertaconazole work well in the current scenario, with systemic antifungals according to each individual case.

The current issue of World Clinics in Dermatology 2019 gives a wide insight into older and newer exciting broad-spectrum topical antifungals.

I hope this edition would be equally helpful to practitioners, dermatology departments and students of dermatology, all over the world.

Rashmi Sarkar MD MNAMS
Professor, Department of Dermatology
Maulana Azad Medical College and Lok Nayak Hospital
New Delhi, India

Email: rashmisarkar@gmail.com

Abbreviations

5FC	5-flucytosine	NCR	Natural coniferous resin
AARS	Aminoacyl tRNA synthetase	Nd:YAG	Neodymium: yttrium-aluminium-garnet
AFST	Antifungal susceptibility testings	NLCs	Nanostructured lipid carriers
AmB	Amphotericin B	OTC	Over-the-counter
BMD	Broth microdilution	PAMP	Pathogen-associated molecular pattern
CC	Clinical cure	PCR	Polymerase chain reaction
CLSI	Clinical and Laboratory Standards Institute	PD	Pharmacodynamics
CoC	Complete cure	PDT	Photodynamic theραpy
DC	Dendritic cell	PK	Pharmacokinetics
DLSO	Distal subungual onychomycosis	POCT	Poivt-of-care testing
DNA	Deoxyribonucleic acid	PRR	Pattern recognition receptor
EPS	Extracellular polymeric substances	PV	Pityriasis versicolor
EUCAST	European Committee on Antimicrobial Susceptibility Testing	RCTs	Randomized controlled trials
FDA	Food and Drug Administration	RFLP	Restriction fragment length polymorphism
HIV	Human immunodeficiency virus	SDD	Susceptible-dose-dependent
IFN-γ	interferon-gamma	SLNs	Solid lipid nanoparticles
IgE	Immunoglobulin E	SQLE	Squalene epoxidase
IH	Immediate hypersensitivity	STI	Sexually transmitted infection
IL-17	Interleukin-17	TCSs	Topical cough suppressants
IL-2	Interleukin-2	Th17	T helper 17
ITS	Internal transcribed spacer	Th1	T helper 1
KOH	Potassium hydroxide	TLR-4	Toll-like receptor 4
LFTs	Liver function tests	TNF-α	Tumor necrosis factor-alpha
MALDI-TOF MS	Matrix-assisted laser desorption/ionization time-of-flight mass spectrometry	TRB	Terbinafine
		tRNA	Transfer ribonucleic acid
		TTO	Tea tree oil
MC	Mycological cure	USFDA	United States Food and Drug Administration
MIC	Minimum inhibitory concentration	UVA	Ultraviolet A
		VVC	Vulvovaginal candidiasis

World Clin Dermatol. 2019;5(1):1-13.

Topical Antifungals and Classes of Topical Antifungal Drugs—An Overview

[1,]*Surabhi Sinha MD DNB MNAMS,
[2]Sidharth Tandon MD, [3]Rashmi Sarkar MD MNAMS

[1]Department of Dermatology and STD, Dr Ram Manohar Lohia Hospital and
Post Graduate Institute of Medical Education Research, New Delhi, India
[2]Consultant Dermatologist, Yashoda Hospital, Ghaziabad, Uttar Pradesh, India
[3]Department of Dermatology, STD and Leprosy, Maulana Azad Medical College and
Lok Nayak Hospital, New Delhi, India

ABSTRACT

Various forms of dermatophytoses have been reported in human population, in both developed and developing countries and an estimated 40 million people suffer from these cutaneous infections. There is a variety of reasons due to which the incidence of dermatophytoses is on the rise; immunosuppression, unscrupulous and unregulated use of over-the-counter topical steroids and change in clothing habits are few of the pertinent ones. Localized infection is usually amenable to topical agents; however, oral antifungal agents may be required for multi-site infection. Various topical antifungal agents have been discussed in detail along with special emphasis on the newer generation antifungal agents.

INTRODUCTION

Dermatophytoses are the most widespread infection amongst the human population with an estimated 40 million people suffering from this cutaneous infection, in developing and underdeveloped countries, in various forms (Figures 1-4).[1] The incidence of dermatophytosis is on the rise because of a variety of reasons—some well-understood and some still under evaluation—

*Corresponding author
Email: surabhi2310@gmail.com

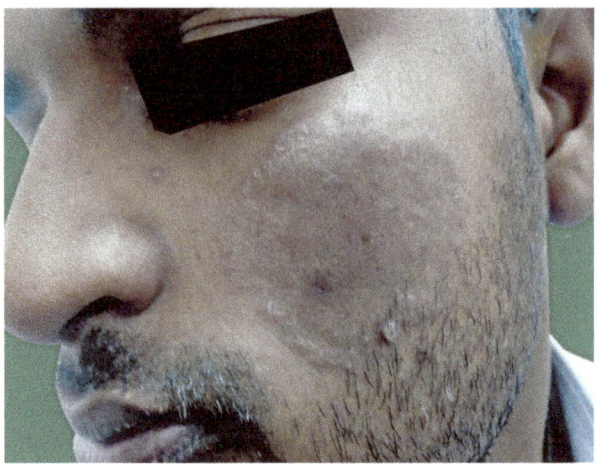

Figure 1: Tinea faciei in adult.

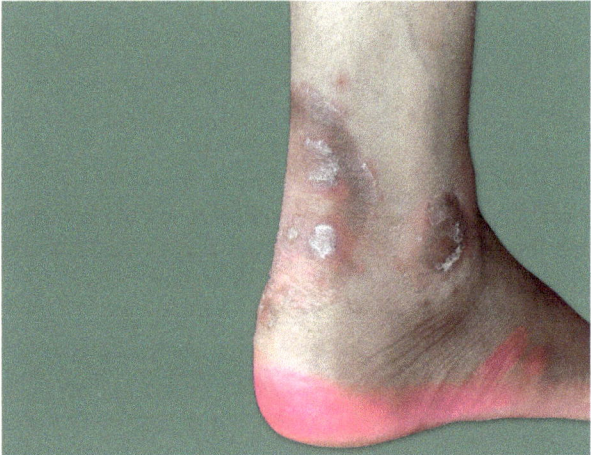

Figure 2: Tinea pedis.

immunosuppression, unscrupulous and unregulated use of over-the-counter topical steroids and change in clothing habits are among the most prominent factors (Figures 5-7).[2]

Antifungal agents can be used both topically and systemically; however, systemic agents are reserved for more widespread or severe fungal infections. Dermatophytoses are usually amenable to topical agents if localized but may need oral antifungals if multisite infection is present or the dermatophytosis is at certain

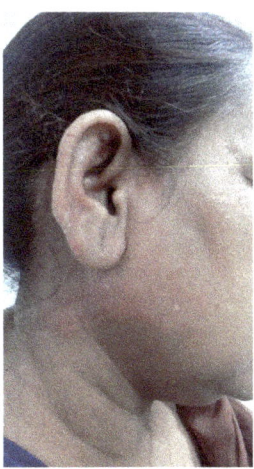

Figure 3: Localized facial tinea in adult which may be amenable to topical antifungal therapy.

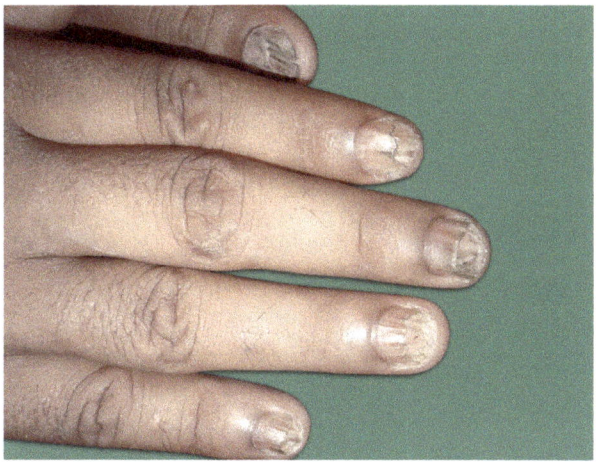

Figure 4: Onychomycosis of all fingernails.

areas like soles, nails, or scalp, etc. Topical treatment of fungal infections took a giant leap in the 1960s when specific antifungal agents were introduced; prior to that, only nonspecific agents were in use, e.g., Castellani's paint, Whitfield's ointment, Gentian violet, potassium permanganate, undecylenic acid and selenium sulfide. Most topical antifungals have to be applied twice daily for long duration but certain newer agents now have the advantage of single application daily and shorter duration of treatment.

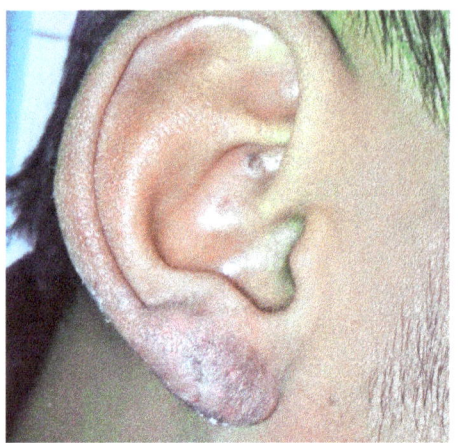

Figure 5: Atypical tinea—Tinea faciei involving unilateral ear lobe.

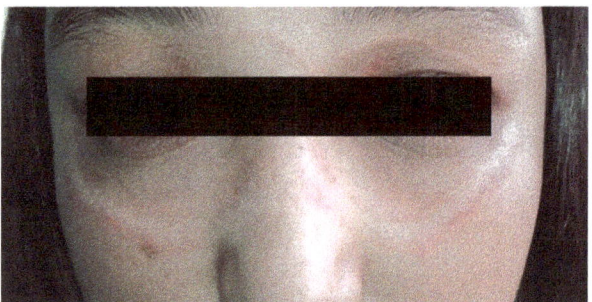

Figure 6: Tinea faciei involving periocular area.

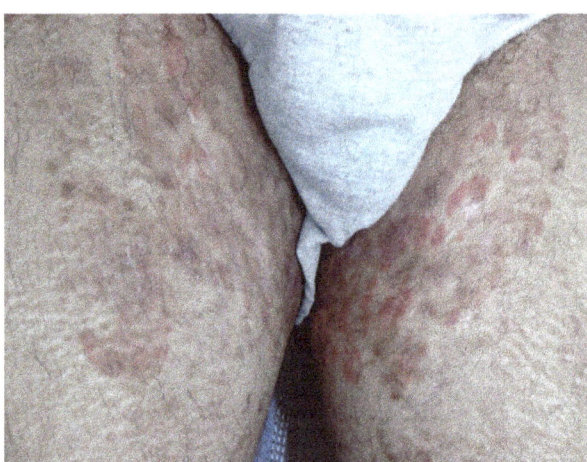

Figure 7: Steroid damage with tinea.

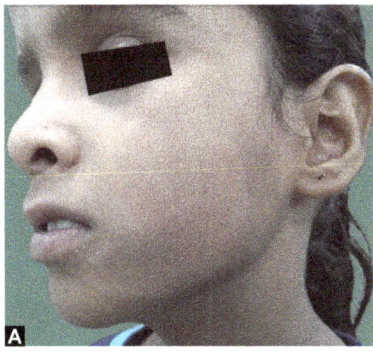 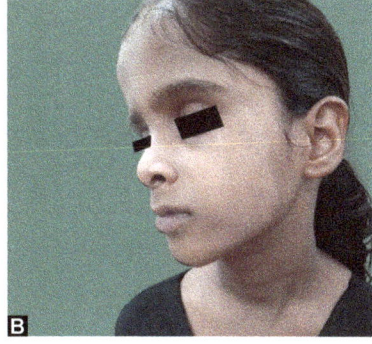

Figure 8: A, Pre-treatment tinea faciei in a child; **B,** Post-treatment improvement in tinea faciei with topical antifungals.

INDICATIONS OF TOPICAL ANTIFUNGALS

Localized dermatophytic infection was previously the main indication of topical antifungal therapy but other important indications include:

* Pregnancy and lactation
* Pediatric dermatophytic infections, especially infants (Figure 8)
* Patients with systemic diseases such as liver, renal or cardiovascular diseases
* Patients on other drugs, which have potential interactions with oral antifungals
* As an adjuvant to systemic therapy
* As adjunctive to systemic therapy
* Prophylactic use to avoid recurrences after adequate oral treatment
* Attempts to shorten, limit or improve systemic antifungal treatment.[3]

CLASSIFICATION OF TOPICAL ANTIFUNGALS[3]

The classification of topical antifungals has been shown in Table 1.

Table 1: Classification of Topical Antifungals	
Azoles: Imidazole	Clotrimazole, miconazole, eberconazole, econazole, ketoconazole, bifonazole, sertaconazole, luliconazole, oxiconazole, tioconazole
Azoles: Triazoles	Fluconazole
Allylamine	Terbinafine
Hydroxypyridones	Ciclopirox
Polyene antibiotics	Amphotericin B
Oxaboroles	Tavaborole
Morpholines	Amorolfine
Others	Tolnaftate
Nonspecific agents	Whitfield's ointment Castellani's paint

MECHANISMS OF ACTION OF
VARIOUS ANTIFUNGAL AGENTS

Azoles

This group comprises of two chemically related subgroups which are imidazoles and triazoles. Triazoles have three nitrogen atoms whereas imidazoles have only two atoms in the azole ring.[4]

The azoles act by inhibition of lanosterol 14α-demethylase of the ergosterol synthesis pathway. This results in the inhibition of conversion of lanosterol to ergosterol. Decreased availability of ergosterol and accumulation of intracellular 14α-methyl sterols result in increased membrane rigidity, increased permeability, and death.

Some of the topical azoles commonly being used nowadays are discussed below:

Eberconazole {1-[2,4-dichloro-10,11-dihydro-5H-dibenzo(a,d)cyclohepten-5-yl]-1H-imidazole} with a molecular formula $C_{18}-H_{14}-C_{12}-N_2$, is a broad-spectrum antifungal agent active against dermatophytes, *Candida*, *Malassezia furfur* and gram-positive bacteria.[5]

It has anti-inflammatory affect akin to aspirin as it can inhibit 5-5-lipooxygenase and cyclooxygenase-2.[6] Its anti-inflammatory action and efficacy against gram-positive bacteria can add to its efficacy in inflamed cutaneous mycoses and in secondary infections, favoring the regression of inflammatory symptoms and treatment compliance. Bothiraja et al. used ethyl-cellulose microsponges as a means of drug delivery and found that the levels of eberconazole nitrate were four-fold higher in the stratum corneum as compared to the conventional preparation in use.[7] Eberconazole has been marketed as a cream with a characteristic lipophilic-hydrophilic molecular structure for better penetration of fungal cell membrane and prolonged duration of action. The galenic components of this topical azole favor and optimize the drug's action in the skin, fatty acid esters facilitate penetration in the skin and make the cream easy to spread, while polyacrylamides produce a filmogenous effect and facilitate the continuance of the active principle in the skin.

The main side effects observed were mild sensation of coldness and pruritus which resolves on repeated application.[5] Eberconazole has been shown to be as effective as and even superior to terbinafine in trials. It has also been shown to have lower MICs than clotrimazole, ketoconazole and miconazole against dermatophytes as well as *Candida* species, esp. *C. krusei* and *C. glabrata* which are usually resistant to triazoles.

Sertaconazole has a unique benzothiophene ring which enhances its lipophilic ability. This imparts it with the ability to bind to nonsterol lipids thus increasing the permeability and also increases dermal retention of the molecule.[8]

Sertaconazole also inhibits the release of interleukin-2 (IL-2), tumor necrosis factor-α, interferon-α, IL-4 and granulocyte-macrophage colony-stimulating factor, and is also active against gram-positive cocci—thus, responsible for its anti-inflammatory and antibacterial activity. It is also known to kill *Trichomonas vaginalis* in vitro and to inhibit dimorphic transformation of *Candida albicans* into its pathogenic form. Contact allergic dermatitis, burning on application, and skin dryness are the possible side effects. It also has antipruritic activity.[9]

Luliconazole is an R-enantiomer of lanoconazole,[10] has an imidazole moiety incorporated into the ketone dithioacetate structure which results in a high potency against dermatophytes with a minimum inhibitory concentration (MIC) levels for *Trichophyton rubrum* which is 1–4 times lower when compared to terbinafine[10] with a strong in vitro activity against *C. albicans* and *Aspergillus fumigatus*.[3]

Efinaconazole, an emerging triazole effective against dermatophytes, *Candida*, and nondermatophyte molds. Efinaconazole 10% topical solution is used for the topical treatment of toenail onychomycosis caused by *T. rubrum* and *T. mentagrophytes*. It reaches the site of infection by transungual penetration. Efinaconazole has better penetration of the nail bed as compared to ciclopirox and amorolfine (14.3% efinaconazole vs. 0.7% and 1.9% for ciclopirox and amorolfine in keratin suspensions, respectively).[11]

Fenticonazole belongs to the imidazole group and has a broad-spectrum of antimycotic activity against dermatophytes and yeasts. Fenticonazole acts by (1) inhibiting the secretion of protease acid by *C. albicans*; (2) damaging the cytoplasmic membrane; and (3) by blocking cytochrome oxidases and peroxidases. Fenticonazole also has been shown to have antibacterial activity against the bacteria which are associated with superinfected fungal skin and vaginal infections, and antiparasitic action against the protozoan *T. vaginalis*. Therefore, fenticonazole may be an ideal topical alternative to multiagent treatment of mixed infections involving mycotic, bacterial, dermatophyte, and/or *Trichomonas* species. Fenticonazole is the only antifungal to have a single dose dependent suppression of candidal proteinase.

It is well-tolerated topically and the adverse effects most commonly noticed with the application of this drug are burning sensation when applied intravaginally.[12]

Allylamines

Terbinafine and naftifine are the two important drugs of this group. Allylamines inhibit the formation of squalene epoxidase, which is a precursor of lanosterol and involved in the formation of cell membrane. The accumulation of high levels of squalene leads to increased membrane permeability and disruption of cellular organization.[6]

Terbinafine

Terbinafine was discovered in 1983 and is different from its parent compound, naftifine, by the presence of a tert-butylacetylene substitution of the phenyl ring on the side chain of the molecule. This confers an additional increase in oral efficacy and increases the in vitro activity 10–100 times that of naftifine.[13] Topical terbinafine has been approved by the Food and Drug Administration (FDA) for tinea cruris, athlete's foot, and tinea corporis.[6] Choudhary et al. found similar efficacy and side effect profile of 1% terbinafine cream as compared to 1% eberconazole nitrate cream in the management of localized tinea cruris and corporis.[14] Terbinafine is also available in newer formulations as transferosome, liposome, liposome film, microemulsion gel, liposome poloxamer gel, liposome ethosome, etc.[15]

Naftifine

Naftifine, a topical allylamine is effective against dermatophytes, *Candida*, *Aspergillus* as well as gram-negative and gram-positive bacteria. Naftifine also acts as an anti-inflammatory agent by blocking the prostaglandin pathway.[16] Naftifine 2% gel has been recommended as a treatment for moccasin type tinea pedis by recently conducted randomized controlled trials (RCTs).[17] FDA has also approved 2% naftifine cream/gel application once daily for 2 weeks, for the treatment of interdigital tinea pedis, tinea cruris, and tinea corporis caused by *T. rubrum* species.[6]

Butenafine

Butenafine is a benzylamine derivative and has potent fungicidal activity against *Aspergillus*, dermatophytes, dimorphic, and dematiaceous fungi with its mechanism of action being similar to the other allylamines. Das et al. found superior efficacy of 1% butenafine cream as compared with 1% terbinafine cream in the treatment of tinea cruris.[18] Thaker et al. in a recently conducted RCT found topical 1% butenafine to be more efficacious and equally safe as compared to 2% sertaconazole for the treatment of tinea infections.[19]

Polyene Antibiotics

Amphotericin B is a broad-spectrum antifungal agent that has been used parenterally. It is still "go to" drug for treatment of disseminated invasive mycoses. It is fungicidal and has a unique structure characterized by both hydrophilic (polyhydroxyl) and hydrophobic (polyene) faces on its long axis. It binds with the ergosterol moiety, forming pores which lead to leakage of monovalent ions (K^+, Na^+, H^+, and Cl^-) and fungal cell death. Topical formulations of amphotericin B have been studied in cutaneous candidiasis and nondermatophyte mold infections and have been found to be efficacious. There have not been many studies on the use of this drug in dermatophytosis in vivo but a handful of studies in vitro have shown encouraging results.[20]

Hydroxypyridones

This class of topical antifungal agents has been described as weak acids with broad-spectrum of antimicrobial activity, which is conferred as a result of its unique mechanism of action which is by chelation of trivalent metal cations leading to the inhibition of metal dependent enzymes. This also explains the low level of resistance which has been reported against these agents.[21] Ciclopirox, octopirox, and rilopirox are the drugs belonging to this class with ciclopirox being the prototype. Various newer formulations of ciclopirox are available which include lipid diffusion enhancers, isopropyl alcohol, urea, potassium hydroxide and have led to increased permeability and efficacy of the drug in the management of onychomycosis.[6]

Morpholines

Morpholines act by inhibition of two enzymes, i.e., C-14 sterol reductase and C-8 sterol isomerase, in the pathway for ergosterol synthesis.

Amorolfine is a phenylpropyl-morpholine derivative and is structurally distinct from other commercially available antifungals. Chemically amorolfine ($C_{21}H_{35}NO$) is cis-4-{3-[4-(1,1-dimethylpropyl)-phenyl]-2-methylpropyl}-2,6-dimethylmorpholine.[22] It has been mainly used for the treatment of onychomycosis in a lacquer formulation with its efficacy and safety being comparable to various azoles.[6]

Oxaboroles

These are a newer class of antifungal agents, which act by blocking protein synthesis by inhibiting leucylaminoacyl transfer RNA (tRNA) synthetase.[23]

Tavaborole was the first oxaborole and was approved by the FDA in 2014 for the treatment of toenail onychomycosis. Its selectivity for fungal aminoacyl tRNA synthetase (AARS) is 1,000 times more as compared to mammalian AARS. The molecular weight of tavaborole is 152 kDa.[6] As a result of this low-molecular weight its permeability within the human nail plate is more as compared to the other antifungal agents.[24] Jinna et al. found that 5% tavaborole has a higher penetration than 8% ciclopirox olamine on a cadaveric nail.[25]

In a meta-analysis of topical antifungals conducted by Rotta et al., it was concluded that all topical antifungals are better than placebos in treatment of localized dermatophytic infections and there was no statistical difference in the efficacy of azoles versus other antifungal agents.[26] However, the mycological cure rates did favor the nonallylamine antifungals but the difference was not statistically significant. Furthermore, it was concluded that azoles are more costeffective as compared to allylamines, and hence, were recommended as first-line antifungal agents with allylamines as the second-line agents in case of failure of azoles.[26]

The adverse events most commonly reported by patients were burning, stinging, and itching, all confined to the site of application and it was difficult to conclude whether they were actual adverse events related to the application of topical antifungals or were just the manifestations of the disease per se.[26]

NEWER TOPICAL FORMULATIONS

The molecular weight of the topical antifungal agent as well as its rate of release from the stratum corneum has led to the development of several carriers for these agents.[27] Some of them are enlisted below.

Micelle

It is defined as a surfactant dispersed in a liquid with the hydrophilic head aligned toward water and the hydrophobic tail sequestered toward inside. Clotrimazole, fluconazole, and econazole have micellar solutions for the treatment of superficial fungal infections.[28]

Microemulsion

A mixture of oil and water stabilized by a surfactant with sizes in nanometer range.

Ketoconazole, itraconazole, voriconazole, econazole and fluconazole have been used as microemulsion gels with enhanced percutaneous absorption.[27]

VESICULAR DRUG DELIVERY UNITS

Vesicles are an assembly of lipid layers which act as depot formulations for the drug in the stratum corneum and also decrease the systemic absorption of the topically applied agent.

These also act in increasing the penetration of the drug into the epidermis as they are lipid soluble.

Liposomes, ethosomes, niosomes, transferosomes and penetration enhancer vesicles are different types of vesicular drug delivery units.[27]

Liposomes

Liposomes are vesicles made of concentric lipid bilayers separated by water or aqueous buffer compartments, ranging in size from 10 nm to 20 µm. Liposomes are either adsorbed onto the skin surface or they may also penetrate via the lipid-rich channels.[27] They can also form occlusive films leading to an increase in skin hydration and drug penetration into the stratum corneum. Liposomal formulations of ketoconazole and ciclopirox olamine have been found to be more efficacious than the conventional preparations.[29]

Transferosomes

These have been defined as deformable liposomes and have phospholoipids and an edge activator as their constituents. The edge activator is a surfactant, which can deform the phospholipid layer, and thus, imparts the transferosome the ability to penetrate deeper layers of the skin. Griseofulvin transferosomes have a higher efficacy in treating dermatophyte infection and amphotericin B has also been used topically as a transferosome.[27]

Ethosomes

These are vesicles which contain ethanol in place of edge activator and the ethanol acts as a penetration enhancer. Ethosomal preparations of clotrimazole and econazole have been used and have been found to be more effective than the liposomal preparations against *Candida*.[27]

Niosomes

These are very similar to liposomes but have nonionic surfactants in place of phospholipids. Griseofulvin and ketoconazole have shown enhanced cure rates in niosomal formulations.[27] Eberconazole too is available as stable nano particles in niosomal gel formulations for better drug delivery.

Penetration Enhancer Vesicles

These are elastic vesicular systems made from soybean lecithin and can penetrate into the deeper layers of the skin. The commonly used penetration enhancers are oleic acid, Labrasol and Transcutol.[27]

SOLID LIPID NANOPARTICLES

The drug is entrapped in a solid lipid core made up of triglycerides, di- and monoglycerides, fatty acids, sterols and waxes.[27]

CONCLUSION

Topical antifungals have limited but important indications. Although, the older azoles have been there for long, newer ones like luliconazole, eberconazole and sertaconazole work well in the current scenario, with systemic antifungals according to each individual case.

REFERENCES

1. Verma S, Madhu R. The great Indian epidemic of superficial dermatophytosis: an appraisal. *Indian J Dermatol.* 2017;62(3):227-36.
2. Rotta I, Otuki MF, Sanches AC, Correr CJ. Efficacy of topical antifungal drugs in different dermatomycoses: a systematic review with meta-analysis. *Rev Assoc Med Bras.* 2012;58(3):308-18.
3. Poojary SA. Topical antifungals: a review and their role in current management of dermatophytoses. *Clin Dermatol Rev.* 2017;1(3):24-9.
4. Zhang AY, Camp WL, Elewski BE. Advances in topical and systemic antifungals. *Dermatol Clin.* 2007;25(2):165-83, vi.
5. Moodahadu-Bangera LS, Martis J, Mittal R, et al. Eberconazole–Pharmacological and clinical review. Indian J Dermatol Venereol Leprol. 2012;78:217-22.
6. Sahni K, Singh S, Dogra S. Newer Topical Treatments in Skin and Nail Dermatophyte Infections. *Indian Dermatol Online J.* 2018;9:149–58.
7. Bothiraja C, Gholap AD, Shaikh KS, Pawar AP. Investigation of ethyl cellulose microsponge gel for topical delivery of eberconazole nitrate for fungal therapy. *Ther Deliv.* 2014;5:781-94.
8. Croxtall JD, Plosker GL. Sertaconazole: a review of its use in the management of superficial mycoses in dermatology and gynaecology. *Drugs.* 2009;69(3):339-59.
9. Liebel F, Lyte P, Garay M, Southall MD. Anti-inflammatory and anti-itch activity of sertaconazole nitrate. *Arch Dermatol Res.* 2006;298(4):191-9.
10. Saunders J, Maki K, Koski R, Nybo SE. Tavaborole, efinaconazole, and luliconazole: three new antimycotic agents for the treatment of dermatophytic fungi. *J Pharm Pract.* 2016;30(6):621-30.
11. Lipner SR, Scher RK. Efinaconazole in the treatment of onychomycosis. *Infect Drug Resist.* 2015;8:163-72.
12. Veraldi S, Milani R. Topical fenticonazole in dermatology and gynaecology. current role in therapy. *Drugs.* 2008;68(15):2183-94.
13. Newland JG, Abdel-Rahman SM. Update on terbinafine with a focus on dermatophytoses. *Clin Cosmet Investig Dermatol.* 2009;2:49-63.
14. Choudhary SV, Aghi T, Bisati S. Efficacy and safety of terbinafine hydrochloride 1% cream vs eberconazole nitrate 1% cream in localised tinea corporis and tinea cruris. *Indian Dermatol Online J.* 2014;5(2):128-31.
15. Tanrıverdi ST, Hilmioğlu Polat S, Yeşim Metin D, Kandiloglu G, Özer Ö. Terbinafine hydrochloride loaded liposome film formulation for treatment of onychomycosis: in vitro and in vivo evaluation. *J Liposome Res.* 2016;26(2):163-73.
16. Gupta AK, Ryder JE, Cooper EA. Naftifine: a review. *J Cutan Med Surg.* 2008;12(2):51-8.
17. Stein Gold LF, Vlahovic T, Verma A, Olayinka B, Fleischer AB Jr. Naftifine hydrochloride gel 2%: an effective topical treatment for moccasin-type tinea pedis. *J Drugs Dermatol.* 2015;14(10):1138-44.

18. Das S, Barbhuniya JN, Biswas I, Bhattacharya S, Kundu PK. Studies on comparison of the efficacy of terbinafine 1% cream and butenafine 1% cream for the treatment of Tinea cruris. *Indian Dermatol Online J.* 2010;1(1):8-9.
19. Thaker SJ, Mehta DS, Shah HA, Dave JN, Mundhava SG. A comparative randomized open label study to evaluate efficacy, safety and cost effectiveness between topical 2% sertaconazole and topical 1% butenafine in tinea infections of skin. *Indian J Dermatol.* 2013;58(6):451-6.
20. Sinha S, Sardana K. Antifungal efficacy of amphotericin B against dermatophytes and its relevance in recalcitrant dermatophytoses: a commentary. *Indian Dermatol Online J.* 2018;9(2):120-2.
21. Subissi A, Monti D, Togni G, Mailland F. Ciclopirox: recent nonclinical and clinical data relevant to its use as a topical antimycotic agent. *Drugs.* 2010;70(16):2133-52.
22. Polak A, Jäckel A, Noack A, Kappe R. Agar sublimation test for the in vitro determination of the antifungal activity of morpholine derivatives. *Mycoses.* 2004;47(5-6):184-92.
23. Poulakos M, Grace Y, Machin JD, Dorval E. Efinaconazole and tavaborole. *J Pharm Pract.* 2017;30(2):245-55.
24. Zane LT, Chanda S, Coronado D, Del Rosso J. Antifungal agents for onychomycosis: new treatment strategies to improve safety. *Dermatol Online J.* 2016;22(3). pii: 13030/qt8dg124gs.
25. Jinna S, Finch J. Spotlight on tavaborole for the treatment of onychomycosis. *Drug Des Devel Ther.* 2015;9:6185-90.
26. Rotta I, Sanchez A, Gonçalves PR, Otuki MF, Correr CJ. Efficacy and safety of topical antifungals in the treatment of dermatomycosis: a systematic review. *Br J Dermatol.* 2012;166(5):927-33.
27. Bseiso EA, Nasr M, Sammour O, Abd El Gawad NA. Recent advances in topical formulation carriers of antifungal agents. *Indian J Dermatol Venereol Leprol.* 2015;81(5):457-63.
28. Bachhav YG, Mondon K, Kalia YN, Gurny R, Möller M. Novel micelle formulations to increase cutaneous bioavailability of azole antifungals. *J Control Release.* 2011;153(2):126-32.
29. Verma A, Palani S. Development and in-vitro evaluation of liposomal gel of ciclopirox olamine. *Int J Pharm Biol Sci.* 2010;1:1-6.

World Clin Dermatol. 2019;5(1):14-28.

Dermatophytoses—What is New?

Sheetanshu Kumar MD, *Vinay Keshavamurthy MD DNB MRCP MNAMS

Department of Dermatology, Venereology and Leprology
Postgraduate Institute of Medical Education and Research, Chandigarh, Punjab, India

ABSTRACT

There is a recently observed ominous shift in the status of dermatophytosis worldwide, especially in India owing to rise in overall prevalence as well as emergence of chronic, recurrent, recalcitrant and resistant dermatophytosis necessitating changes in treatment protocol and diagnostic modalities. The observed change in clinico-epidemiological trend can be attributed to several factors like overcrowding, rapid urbanization, poor hygiene, rise in number of immunosuppressed hosts due to diabetes, human immuno-deficiency virus (HIV), immunosuppressive medications and most importantly rampant misuse of topical steroids and freely available unholy combination of topical corticosteroid-antibacterial-antifungal. While previously *Trichophyton rubrum* was known to be the most common species causing dermatophytosis, recent studies have suggested the shift from *T. rubrum* to *Trichophyton mentagrophytes* as the most common causative organism of dermatophytosis. This is coupled with changes in clinical presentation with rise in proportion of atypical presentations.

There are also newer insights into the pathogenesis of dermatophytosis suggesting a role of T helper 17 (Th17) pathway in immunity against dermatophytosis and role of biofilms in resistance against antifungals. Diagnostic and treatment modalities have evolved with introduction of molecular methods like polymerase chain reaction (PCR) in diagnosis and newer treatment modalities like photodynamic therapy and lasers in treatment.

*Corresponding author
Email: vinay.keshavmurthy@gmail.com

INTRODUCTION

Superficial fungal infections are estimated to affect 20–25% of population of world in their lifetime.[1] Dermatophytosis is a subtype of superficial fungal infection caused by invasion of keratinized tissue like skin, hair and nails by dermatophytes usually of the genera *Trichophyton*, *Epidermophyton*, or *Microsporum*. In a study from south India, dermatophytosis accounted for approximately 30–40% of patient load of dermatology outpatient departments of various medical colleges.[2]

The extent of dermatophytosis may range from mild or localized to severe or extensive depending upon the host's immune response to the microorganism and other environmental factors. Previously 80% of patients developing acute dermatophytosis were known to respond to standard antifungal treatment while about 20% developed chronic dermatophytosis exhibiting poor response to antifungal agents.[3] However, the scenario of dermatophytosis in India and worldwide is changing rapidly owing to major epidemiological shifts and emergence of recalcitrant and resistant dermatophytosis necessitating changes in treatment protocol and diagnostic modalities.[4] In this article, we will be discussing the recent trends in epidemiology, newer insights into pathogenesis and clinical features of dermatophytosis as well as newer developments in diagnosis and treatment.

RECENT TRENDS IN EPIDEMIOLOGY

A significant shift in the epidemiology of dermatophytosis is being observed recently with increase in the overall prevalence of dermatophytosis along with a substantial surge in the recalcitrant, recurrent and extensive dermatophytosis (Figure 1). Worldwide *T. rubrum* was found to be the most common cause of dermatophytic infections followed by *T. mentagrophytes*.[5] However, recent studies from India have detected the shift of most common causative pathogen of dermatophytosis from *T. rubrum* to *T. mentagrophytes* especially in past 3–4 years.[4] The factors contributing to the higher incidence of dermatophytosis and recent shift in clinico-epidemiology include overcrowding, poverty, poor hygiene, contact with animals,[6] hot and humid climate,[1] occupations which require working in hot and humid conditions,[7] recent changes in attire and dressing sense like increased use of tight-fitting garments of synthetic fibers and occlusive footwear and rise in number of immunosuppressed hosts due to diabetes, HIV, immunosuppressive medications. Another major factor contributing to this epidemic is the rampant misuse of topical steroids and freely available combination of topical corticosteroid-antibacterial-antifungal which is being prescribed as panacea for all the dermatological conditions by general practitioners, alternative medicine practitioners and "chemists" and also being self-medicated by the patients.[8]

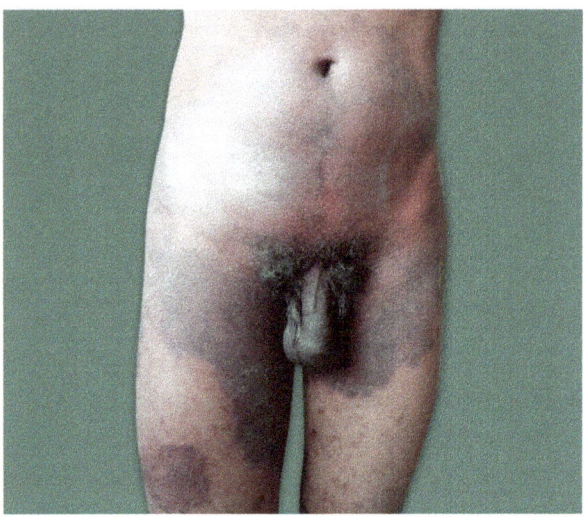

Figure 1: Extensive tinea corporis and cruris.

Rise in Incidence of Chronic and Recurrent Dermatophytosis

Although the terms chronic dermatophytosis and recurrent dermatophytosis are used very commonly, consensus regarding standard definition for these terms are lacking. These terms have been defined on the basis of duration of disease or according to the response to treatment. Chronic dermatophytosis was defined by Hay et al.[9] in 1982 as "dermatophytosis which has not responded to topical or systemic antifungal therapy and runs a chronic course with episodic periods of remission".[9] On the basis of duration, chronic dermatophytosis has been defined arbitrarily as "patients who have suffered from the disease for more than 6 months to 12 months, with or without recurrence, despite adequate treatment".[10] The term "recurrent dermatophytosis" has been defined as "dermatophytic infection which runs a protracted course with phases of remission and exacerbation".[11] Recurrent or chronic dermatophytosis has emerged as a challenging health problem in India in last few years having significant financial and psychosocial implications on the patient and the society.[12] Exact prevalence of chronic and recurrent dermatophytosis in India is not known, but it was found to vary between 5 and 10% in different studies.[10] The prevalence of recurrent dermatophytosis was found to be 9.3% in a recent study by Pathania et al.[13] The major recent epidemiological studies on dermatophytosis including recurrent and chronic dermatophytosis have been summarized in Table 1.

Table 1: Major Recent Indian Studies on Dermatophytosis including Recurrent and Chronic Dermatophytosis

Author (year)	Type of study	Location	Most common causative species	Most common clinical type	KOH positivity	Culture positivity	Other salient findings
Sharma et al. (2017)[14]	Clinico-epidemiological study on recurrent dermatophytosis	Sikkim, India	T. mentagrophytes (40%), T. schoenleinii (33.3%), T. tonsurans (16.6%), T. rubrum (6.6%)	Tinea corporis (54.16%) followed by tinea unguium (15.63%)	55.2%	63.5%	Recurrence rate—34.3% Clinical cure rate—58.3%
Mahajan et al. (2017)[15]	Clinico-mycological study on dermatophytosis	Varanasi, India	T. mentagrophytes (75.9%), T. rubrum (21.9%), T. tonsurans (0.7%)	Tinea corporis and cruris (27.2%)	79.6%	52.4%	Itraconazole found to be the most effective drug, followed by ketoconazole, terbinafine and fluconazole. Griseofulvin—least effective drug
Dabas et al. (2017)[16]	Clinico-mycological and molecular (species distribution and susceptibility pattern) study on dermatophytosis	New Delhi, India	T. interdigitale (mentagrophytes)—56%, T. tonsurans (25.7%), T. rubrum (7.5%)	Tinea cruris (37.9%) followed by tinea corporis (29%)	74.1%	53.2%	High MIC values were observed for T. tonsurans and T. rubrum to terbinafine and griseofulvin
Rudramurthy et al. (2017)[17]	Mutation study evaluating drug resistance	Chandigarh, India	T. interdigitale (66.1%), T. rubrum (26.3%), T. tonsurans (3%), M. gypseum (3%)	Tinea corporis (30.2%), tinea cruris (28.2%)	-	-	T1189C mutation in squalene epoxide gene resulting in Phe397Leu substitution in almost one-quarter of isolates of the terbinafine having high MICs suggests it as one of the probable mechanisms of terbinafine resistance
Pathania et al. (2018)[13]	Clinico-epidemiological study on recurrent dermatophytosis	Chandigarh, India	T. mentagrophytes (40%) followed by T. rubrum (32.2%)	Mixed (64.6%) followed by tinea cruris (17.3%), tinea corporis (18%)	98.7%	60%	MIC was lowest for itraconazole followed by terbinafine, fluconazole and griseofulvin
Nenoff et al. (2018)[4]	Molecular study	India—multicentric	T. mentagrophytes (93.2%) followed by T. rubrum (6.8%)	Tinea corporis (65.6%), tinea cruris (28.8%)	-	74.1%	Marked and dramatic shift of causative species of dermatophytosis from T. rubrum to T. mentagrophytes

Rise in Incidence of Deep Dermatophytosis

Deep dermatophytosis is seen due to deeper invasion by dermatophytic strains, usually presenting clinically as nodular asymptomatic lesions with occasional overlying skin ulceration. Physical barriers like epidermal keratin, rapid turnover of keratinocytes, skin pH, fatty acids secreted by sebaceous glands generally prevents the deeper penetration of dermatophytes. Deep dermatophytosis is seen usually in individuals who are either immunosuppressed or have impaired physical barrier. There has been increase in the incidence of deep dermatophytosis as well owing to the rising population of immunocompromised hosts. In a report by Lanternier et al.,[18] it was observed that *CARD9* gene mutation was associated with deep dermatophytosis in a North African family.[18]

NEWER INSIGHTS INTO PATHOGENESIS OF DERMATOPHYTOSIS

Role of Th17 Pathway in Pathogenesis of Dermatophytosis

Contrary to the previous knowledge that Th1 immune pathway is solely responsible for immunity against dermatophytosis, newer studies have pointed toward the involvement of Th17 pathway in immunity against dermatophytosis.[19] A mouse model study by Nakamura et al.[20] found that application of *Trichophyton* antigen known as trichophytin leads to induction of both Th1 and Th17 cells. Sakuragi et al.[21] also observed increased Th17 cells in peripheral blood of a patient suffering from tinea capitis further suggesting the role of Th17 pathway in immunity against dermatophytosis. Loss of Th17 cell function has also been found to be associated with higher chances of dermatophytosis.[19] In their study on mouse model, Burstein et al.[22] also found the role of Th17 pathway and neutrophil recruitment in dermatophytosis limited to epidermis. They also concluded that absence of a functional interleukin-17 (IL-17) pathway leads to colonization of epidermis by dermatophytes.[22]

Pathogenesis of Chronic and Recurrent Dermatophytosis

There is paucity of literature regarding the pathogenesis of chronic and resistant dermatophytosis. Different studies on chronic dermatophytosis have attributed defective Th2 immunity and failure in patients to mount adequate cell-mediated immune response as factors leading to development of chronic dermatophytosis. In a recent study by De Sousa et al.,[23] patients suffering from chronic and widespread *T. rubrum* infection were found to have immunological defects involving impaired release of free radicals and nitric oxide along with dysfunctional macrophage killing mechanisms.[23,24] Rand et al.[25] found that atopic patients are more susceptible to chronic dermatophytosis probably owing to antagonizing actions of cell-mediated immunity and humoral immunity.[9,25] Patients suffering from chronic and recurrent dermatophytosis are also usually found to be resistant to standard antifungal treatment. Also, inadequate doses or duration of antifungal drugs may lead to improper eradication of infection further leading to chronic or recurrent infections.[10]

EMERGING DRUG RESISTANCE IN DERMATOPHYTOSIS

Several host and microbial factors like indiscriminate use of antifungals especially in inadequate doses or duration, use of topical steroids, rise in the number of immunosuppressed hosts, genetic mutation in dermatophytes, structural alteration of target protein, decreased uptake and increased efflux of drug play a role in emerging antifungal drug resistance.[26]

Clinical resistance is defined as the failure to cure a fungal infection despite the administration of adequate doses of antifungal drug with in vitro activity against the fungus. Microbiological resistance refers to nonsusceptibility of a fungus in in vitro susceptibility testing to a particular antifungal agent when minimum inhibitory concentration (MIC) of the drug exceeds the susceptibility breakpoint for that organism.[26] MIC values of antifungal drugs were found to be higher in Indian patients as compared to western data in a cross-sectional study by Sardana et al.[27] in 40 patients with recalcitrant dermatophytosis. The major mechanisms of resistance to various antifungal agents have been summarized in Table 2.

Biofilms are being recognized as a new mechanism adopted by dermatophytes for development of antifungal drug resistance. Biofilms are formed by the secretion of extracellular matrix encasing entire microbial community after adhering to a foreign substrate. Toukabri et al.[29] assessed the in vitro ability of dermatophyte species causing foot mycosis in forming biofilms and the ability of antifungal agents to prevent its formation. While all dermatophyte species possessed the ability to form biofilm, terbinafine was the most effective agent in prevention of biofilm formation.[29] Brilhante et al.[30] found that *T. rubrum*, *Microsporum gypseum* and *Trichophyton tonsurans* possessed the ability to form strong biofilm while *Microsporum canis* was found to produce weakest biofilm.[30]

Another factor contributing to the problem of drug resistance is the rampant use of substandard formulations of systemic and topical antifungal agents in India due to lack of strict regulation and quality control regarding the manufacturing of drugs. Many of the antifungal brands available commercially do not adhere to the guidelines regarding the manufacturing of drugs, but are nevertheless sold rampantly due to dubious marketing among the chemists and clinicians both. Most of the times, chemists substitute the authentic prescribed brands by the

Table 2: Mechanisms of Resistance of Different Antifungal Drugs[28]	
Drugs	**Mechanism of resistance**
Terbinafine	• Modification of target enzyme by mutation • Increased drug efflux • Stress adaptation • Overexpression of salicylate monooxygenase
Fluconazole	• Increased drug efflux • Stress adaptation
Itraconazole	• Increased drug efflux
Ketoconazole	• Increased drug efflux • Overexpression of lanosterol 14-demethylase
Imazalil	• Increased drug efflux
Tioconazole	• Increased drug efflux • Stress adaptation
Amphotericin B	• Increased drug efflux • Stress adaptation
Griseofulvin	• Increased drug efflux • Stress adaptation

clinicians with these substandard antifungal brands, a practice which is very common and unfortunately not recognized by uneducated or even well-educated patients. These poor quality antifungal brands with questionable pharmacokinetics further accentuating the risk of resistance.

CHANGES IN CLINICAL PRESENTATIONS

Apart from usual clinical presentations of dermatophytosis, there has been recent increase in the atypical presentations of dermatophytosis due to several factors. Several morphological features characterize atypical dermatophytosis which include severe inflammatory lesions with ill-demarcated borders, scaling in the center instead of central clearing, along with follicular papules, vesicles or pustules associated with induration or hyperpigmentation occasionally. Term "tinea incognito" was coined by Ive and Marks to represent lesions of dermatophytosis whose clinical presentation have been modified by the use of topical steroids.[31] Tinea pseudoimbricata[32] is a form of tinea incognito characterized clinically by two or rarely three concentric circles within a lesion of dermatophytosis. Presence of tinea pseudoimbricata is a clue pointing toward the application of potent topical corticosteroid preparations. It resembles tinea imbricata caused by *Trichophyton concentricum*, which is characterized by multiple concentric rings and generalized distribution as compared to pseudoimbricata. Familial forms of dermatophytosis are also being observed recently.[33] Tinea recidivans is seen due to initial response to treatment followed by relapse while on treatment or after stopping treatment. It is characterized by new lesions of dermatophytosis occurring at the periphery of the healing lesions (Figure 2).[34] Several other atypical morphological variants have been described in literature mimicking the lesions of other dermatosis such as erythema multiforme, seborrheic dermatitis, lupus erythematosus, dermatitis herpetiformis, rosacea (Figure 3), eczematous dermatitis (Figure 4), pityriasis rosea, impetigo and polymorphous light eruption.[1] Misuse of topical steroids is one of the major causes of atypical presentations of dermatophytosis along with other factors like resistance and immunosuppressed host.[35]

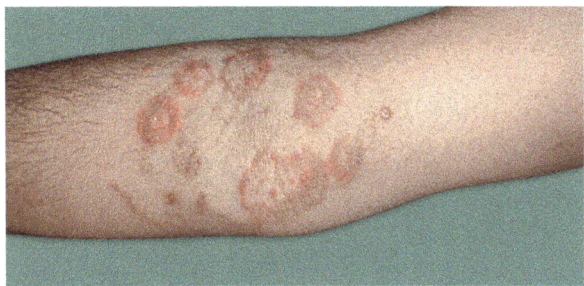

Figure 2: Tinea recidivans: New lesions of dermatophytosis occurring at the periphery of the healing lesions.

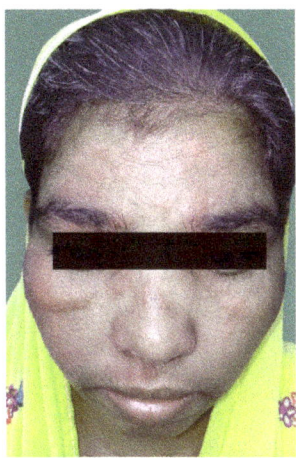

Figure 3: Rosacea-like tinea faciei.

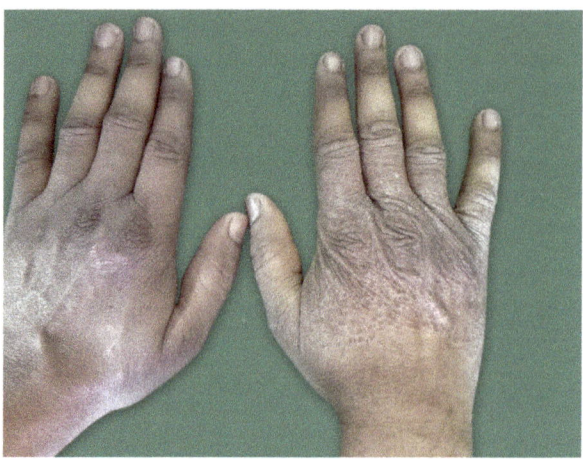

Figure 4: Eczema-like tinea manuum.

RECENT DEVELOPMENTS IN DIAGNOSTIC MODALITIES

Molecular Techniques in Diagnosis of Dermatophytosis

While traditional diagnostic modalities like potassium hydroxide (KOH) mount and culture have remained the backbone of diagnosis of dermatophytosis, molecular techniques have emerged as faster and more accurate diagnostic modality for dermatophytosis with a turnout time of 72 hours or lesser.[36] Molecular methods are also being used for identification of strains whenever identification by conventional methods is not possible. Commonly used molecular methods include PCR—restriction fragment length polymorphism (RFLP), real-time PCR, arbitrarily primed PCR, double-round PCR and PCR-direct sequencing. Deoxyribonucleic acid (DNA) of dermatophytes can also be detected directly in clinical samples. Although they are reliable methods for species identification and differentiation, differentiation of pathogenic from nonpathogenic species cannot be achieved by PCR. For rapid identification of dermatophyte species, matrix-assisted laser desorption/ionization time-of-flight mass spectrometry (MALDI-TOF MS) can also be used.[37] A recent study by Brillowska-Dabrowska et al.[38] assessed the specificity and sensitivity of PCR in identifying the 15 culture proven cases of *M. canis* out of 130 clinical samples. All the 15 cases were identified correctly without any false-positive or false-negative results. However, molecular modalities are expensive and not available widely. Nonetheless, owing to their accuracy, they have a huge potential and widespread use of these modalities are expected in future.

RECENT DEVELOPMENTS IN TREATMENT MODALITIES

Recent Developments in Topical Treatment

Topical antifungal agents are being used both as monotherapy as well as adjuvant to systemic antifungal therapy in treatment of dermatophytosis in extensive disease. A meta-analysis including 65 studies was performed recently by Rotta et al.[39] to compare the efficacy of 14 topical antifungal agents in the treatment of dermatophytosis using a mixed treatment comparison model. No significant difference among the topical antifungal agents was observed with respect to the mycological cure at the end of the treatment. With respect to the sustained cure outcome, butenafine hydrochloride and terbinafine hydrochloride were found to be associated with better outcome as compared to clotrimazole, oxiconazole nitrate, and sertaconazole nitrate. Terbinafine was also found to demonstrate statistical better results as compared to ciclopirox (ciclopirox olamine), and better outcome was observed with naftifine hydrochloride as compared to oxiconazole.[39]

Efinaconazole 10% solution has been emerging as a promising topical modality for treatment of dermatophytosis. A report describing two phase III multicenter trials found mycological cure rate of 53.4% and 55.2% and complete cure rate of 15.2% and 17.8% with once daily application of 10% efinaconazole for 48 weeks in toenail onychomycosis.[40] The mycological cure rate was found to be comparable to oral itraconazole and terbinafine. In a recent study by Noguchi et al., topical 10% efinaconazole was also found to be effective treatment modality in onychomycosis.[41] Being a topical agent, the risk of systemic toxicities is minimal and it can be used in patients where systemic antifungal drugs are contraindicated.

Photodynamic Therapy as an Emerging Modality in Treatment of Dermatophytosis

Amidst the concerns regarding rising resistance to antifungal agents, photo-dynamic therapy (PDT) is emerging as potential treatment option for dermatophytosis.[42] In a comprehensive review by Smijs et al.,[43] several in vitro and ex vivo studies regarding the use of PDT against all the three genera of dermatophytes have been summarized. Various photosensitizers which included 5-aminolevulinic acid, porphyrins, methylene blue, proflavine hemisulfate, etc. were used in these studies. The light sources used in the studies included ultraviolet A (UVA) black light, Oriel solar simulator (Oriel Instruments, Newport Corp, Stratford, CT, USA), and the Paterson lamp (Photo therapeutics, Altrincham, Cheshire, UK). In vitro and ex vivo fungicidal effects were observed with various light sources and photosensitizers.[43] Ex vivo data suggested PDT to be fungicidal against both mature fungal forms and fungal spores. PDT has been used in various reports to treat different forms of dermatophytosis which include onychomycosis, tinea cruris, tinea pedis, etc. caused by different species such as *T. rubrum* or *T. mentagrophytes*. One to four PDT sessions were required usually to clear the infection.[42] Complete mycological cure was achieved in 31 of 59 patients (53%) of dermatophytosis treated with PDT. The treatment refractoriness of onychomycosis to antifungal therapy often requires prolonged systemic therapy with antifungal drugs thus putting the patient at risk to the increased toxicity of antifungal drugs. PDT is a promising therapeutic option especially in patients of onychomycosis in whom prolonged systemic antifungal therapy is not feasible.

Laser Therapy as an Emerging Modality in Treatment of Dermatophytosis

Nonablative laser therapy was recognized as an alternative therapeutic option in the treatment of onychomycosis almost a decade ago. The 1064-nm neodymium:yttrium-aluminum-garnet (Nd:YAG) laser was approved by the Food and Drug Administration (FDA) as a therapeutic modality for treatment of onychomycosis in 2010[44] and currently four types of laser are FDA-approved for the same indication.[45] However, there is still a scarcity of evidence supporting the efficacy of lasers for treatment of onychomycosis.[44] Most of the studies assessing the role of lasers in onychomycosis are small pilot studies or case series/reports. Carney et al. did not observe any improvement in onychomycosis severity score in an in vivo study analyzing the efficacy of five treatments of submillisecond 1064-nm Nd:YAG laser in eight patients with toenail onychomycosis.[46] However, a recent retrospective analysis of 56 patients found 1064-nm diode laser to be an effective treatment modality in the treatment of onychomycosis with positive correlation of treatment efficacy with number of treatment sessions.[44] Nonetheless, role of lasers in onychomycosis treatment still remains controversial.

FUTURE PERSPECTIVES

Retinoids in Dermatophytosis

Ardeshna et al.[47] reported successful treatment of recurrent dermatophytosis in three patients with a combination of isotretinoin and itraconazole. It was hypothesized by the authors that modulation of epidermal growth and cell turnover by retinoids may help in stopping the growth of dermatophytic infection in the epidermis. Currently a randomized controlled trial is going on in a tertiary care center at Chandigarh comparing the combination of isotretinoin and itraconazole/terbinafine with itraconazole/terbinafine in recurrent dermatophytosis.[48]

Vaccines in Dermatophytosis

Although vaccines for immune prophylaxis of dermatophytosis in animals including cattle, horse, dog and cat are available with ongoing attempts to further increase its efficacy,[49] no vaccines for humans exist till date. Immunotherapy and immune prophylaxis against dermatophytosis in humans may be field of interest in future especially in view of recent rise in its incidence and surge in resistant, chronic cases, which are recalcitrant to available treatment modalities.

RECOMMENDATIONS FROM THE RECENT EXPERT CONSENSUS IN INDIA REGARDING THE DIAGNOSIS AND MANAGEMENT OF DERMATOPHYTOSIS[50]

Recently an expert consensus was formulated by 11 experts in the field of dermatology and mycology from India with the help of modified Delphi process comprised of two workshops along with five rounds of questionnaires. The consensus recommended KOH mount and microscopy as the point-of-care test in dermatophytosis while fungal culture should be performed in recurrent, chronic, recalcitrant and extensive dermatophytosis. MALDI-TOF MS was recognized as a promising experimental diagnostic technique but not practical for a real world scenario as it cannot be directly performed on clinical specimens, requiring a mandatory prerequisite of culture. Topical antifungal therapy was recommended for localized cases of naïve tinea cruris and corporis while a combination of systemic and topical antifungal agents was advocated for naïve and recalcitrant lesions of tinea pedis, extensive tinea corporis and recalcitrant tinea cruris and corporis. Topical azoles should be preferred owing to its broad-spectrum activity along with its anti-inflammatory and antibacterial properties. Terbinafine and itraconazole were recommended as the preferred systemic antifungal agents. The recommended minimum duration of treatment was 2–4 weeks in naïve tinea cases and more than 4 weeks in recalcitrant tinea cases. There was a uniform consensus among experts discouraging strongly the use of topical corticosteroids in management of dermatophytosis. Treatment with topical agents was recommended to be continued till 2 weeks after cure while systemic agents after cure should be continued only in recalcitrant cases. Doubling of terbinafine dose (500 mg/day) can be done in cases of recalcitrant tinea while uniform consensus regarding the doubling of itraconazole dose could not be reached. Fluconazole and terbinafine were recommended as the preferred systemic drugs in the pediatric population. Systemic antifungal agents should be avoided in pregnancy and only topical agents should be used.

CONCLUSION

The incidence of dermatophytosis has reached almost to an epidemic level in the recent past owing to factors like overcrowding, rapid urbanization, increase in the number of immunosuppressed hosts, rampant misuse of topical steroids and resistance to antifungal agents. There has also been increase in the cases of chronic, recurrent and recalcitrant cases of dermatophytosis and dermatophytosis presenting with extensive and atypical lesions. The clinicians are also facing the challenge of emerging drug resistance in patients of dermatophytosis due to use of topical steroids and availability of substandard systemic and oral formulations of antifungal agents. Molecular methods like PCR for diagnosis of dermatophytosis are emerging as an accurate and reliable modality, although its use is limited to the experimental setting. PDT and lasers are also emerging as alternative treatment modalities in the treatment of dermatophytosis especially in refractory cases or in cases where systemic antifungal drugs are contraindicated.

REFERENCES

1. Sahoo AK, Mahajan R. Management of tinea corporis, tinea cruris, and tinea pedis: a comprehensive review. *Indian Dermatol Online J.* 2016;7:77-86.
2. Poluri LV, Indugula JP, Kondapaneni SL. Clinicomycological study of dermatophytosis in south India. *J Lab Physicians.* 2015;7:84-9.
3. Blutfield MS, Lohre JM, Pawich DA, Vlahovic TC. The immunologic response to *Trichophyton rubrum* in lower extremity fungal infections. *J Fungi.* 2015;1:130-7.
4. Nenoff P, Verma SB, Vasani R, et al. The current Indian epidemic of superficial dermatophytosis due to *Trichophyton mentagrophytes*: a molecular study. *Mycoses.* 2018.
5. Singh S, Beena P. Profile of dermatophyte infections in Baroda. *Indian J Dermatol Venereol Leprol.* 2003;69:281-3.
6. Qadim HH, Golforoushan F, Azimi H, Goldust M. Factors leading to dermatophytosis. *Ann Parasitol.* 2013;59:99-102.
7. Gurcan S, Tikvesli M, Eskiocak M, Kilic H, Otkun M. Investigation of the agents and risk factors of dermatophytosis: a hospital-based study. *Mikrobiyol Bul.* 2008;42:95-102.
8. Bishnoi A, Narang T, Handa S, et al. Paraneoplastic bullous pemphigoid associated with penile squamous cell carcinoma. *J Eur Acad Dermatol Venereol.* 2018;32:e140-e1.
9. Hay RJ. Chronic dermatophyte infections. I. Clinical and mycological features. *Br J Dermatol.* 1982;106:1-7.
10. Dogra S, Uprety S. The menace of chronic and recurrent dermatophytosis in India: is the problem deeper than we perceive? *Indian Dermatol Online J.* 2016;7:73-6.
11. Sentamilselvi G, Kamalam A, Ajithadas K, Janaki C, Thambiah AS. Scenario of chronic dermatophytosis: an Indian study. *Mycopathologia.* 1997;140:129-35.
12. Ranganathan S, Menon T, Selvi SG, Kamalam A. Effect of socio-economic status on the prevalence of dermatophytosis in Madras. *Indian J Dermatol Venereol Leprol.* 1995;61:16-8.
13. Pathania S, Rudramurthy SM, Narang T, Saikia UN, Dogra S. A prospective study of the epidemiological and clinical patterns of recurrent dermatophytosis at a tertiary care hospital in India. *Indian J Dermatol Venereol Leprol.* 2018;84:678-84.
14. Sharma R, Adhikari L, Sharma RL. Recurrent dermatophytosis: a rising problem in Sikkim, a Himalayan state of India. *Indian J Pathol Microbiol.* 2017;60:541-5.

15. Mahajan S, Tilak R, Kaushal SK, Mishra RN, Pandey SS. Clinico-mycological study of dermatophytic infections and their sensitivity to antifungal drugs in a tertiary care center. *Indian J Dermatol Venereol Leprol*. 2017;83:436-40.

16. Dabas Y, Xess I, Singh G, Pandey M, Meena S. Molecular identification and antifungal susceptibility patterns of clinical dermatophytes following CLSI and EUCAST guidelines. *J Fungi (Basel)*. 2017;3:17.

17. Rudramurthy SM, Shankarnarayan SA, Dogra S, et al. Mutation in the squalene epoxidase gene of *Trichophyton interdigitale* and *Trichophyton rubrum* associated with allylamine resistance. *Antimicrob Agents Chemother*. 2018;62(5). pii: e02522-17.

18. Lanternier F, Pathan S, Vincent QB, et al. Deep dermatophytosis and inherited CARD9 deficiency. *N Engl J Med*. 2013;369:1704-14.

19. Heinen MP, Cambier L, Fievez L, Mignon B. Are Th17 cells playing a role in immunity to dermatophytosis? *Mycopathologia*. 2017;182:251-61.

20. Nakamura T, Nishibu A, Yasoshima M, et al. Analysis of Trichophyton antigen-induced contact hypersensitivity in mouse. *J Dermatol Sci*. 2012;66:144-53.

21. Sakuragi Y, Sawada Y, Hara Y, et al. Increased circulating Th17 cell in a patient with tinea capitis caused by *Microsporum canis*. *Allergol Int*. 2016;65:215-6.

22. Burstein VL, Guasconi L, Beccacece I, et al. IL-17-mediated immunity controls skin infection and T helper 1 response during experimental Microsporum canis dermatophytosis. *J Invest Dermatol*. 2018;138(8):1744-53.

23. de Sousa Mda G, Santana GB, Criado PR, Benard G. Chronic widespread dermatophytosis due to Trichophyton rubrum: a syndrome associated with a Trichophyton-specific functional defect of phagocytes. *Front Microbiol*. 2015;6:801.

24. Almeida SR. Immunology of dermatophytosis. *Mycopathologia*. 2008;166:277-83.

25. Rand HR, Nidhal AM, Rasool D. Atopy as a risk factor for dermatophytoses. *AJPS*. 2005;2(1):25-8.

26. Kanafani ZA, Perfect JR. Resistance to antifungal agents: mechanisms and clinical impact. *Clin Infect Dis*. 2008;46:120-8.

27. Sardana K, Kaur R, Arora P, Goyal R, Ghunawat S. Is antifungal resistance a cause for treatment failure in dermatophytosis: a study focused on tinea corporis and cruris from a tertiary centre? *Indian Dermatol Online J*. 2018;9:90-5.

28. Martinez-Rossi NM, Peres NT, Rossi A. Antifungal resistance mechanisms in dermatophytes. *Mycopathologia*. 2008;166:369-83.

29. Toukabri N, Corpologno S, Bougnoux ME, et al. In vitro biofilms and antifungal susceptibility of dermatophyte and non-dermatophyte moulds involved in foot mycosis. *Mycoses*. 2018;61:79-87.

30. Brilhante RS, Correia EE, Guedes GM, et al. Quantitative and structural analyses of the in vitro and ex vivo biofilm-forming ability of dermatophytes. *J Med Microbiol*. 2017;66:1045-52.

31. Ive FA, Marks R. Tinea incognito. *Br Med J*. 1968;3:149-52.

32. Verma S. Tinea pseudoimbricata. *Indian J Dermatol Venereol Leprol*. 2017;83:344-5.

33. Gazit R, Hershko K, Ingbar A, et al. Immunological assessment of familial tinea corporis. *J Eur Acad Dermatol Venereol*. 2008;22:871-4.

34. Dogra S, Narang T. Emerging atypical and unusual presentations of dermatophytosis in India. *Clin Dermatol Rev*. 2017;1:12-8.

35. Verma S, Madhu R. The great Indian epidemic of superficial dermatophytosis: an appraisal. *Indian J Dermatol*. 2017;62:227-36.

36. Jensen RH, Arendrup MC. Molecular diagnosis of dermatophyte infections. *Curr Opin Infect Dis*. 2012;25:126-34.

37. Verrier J, Monod M. Diagnosis of dermatophytosis using molecular biology. *Mycopathologia*. 2017;182:193-202.

38. Brillowska-Dabrowska A, Michalek E, Saunte DM, Nielsen SS, Arendrup MC. PCR test for *Microsporum canis* identification. *Med Mycol*. 2013;51:576-9.

39. Rotta I, Ziegelmann PK, Otuki MF, et al. Efficacy of topical antifungals in the treatment of dermatophytosis: a mixed-treatment comparison meta-analysis involving 14 treatments. *JAMA Dermatol*. 2013;149:341-9.

40. Elewski BE, Rich P, Pollak R, et al. Efinaconazole 10% solution in the treatment of toenail onychomycosis: two phase III multicenter, randomized, double-blind studies. *J Am Acad Dermatol*. 2013;68:600-8.

41. Noguchi H, Matsumoto T, Hiruma M, et al. Topical efinaconazole: a promising therapeutic medication for tinea unguium. *J Dermatol*. 2018;45:1225-8.

42. Laniosz V, Wetter DA. What's new in the treatment and diagnosis of dermatophytosis? *Semin Cutan Med Surg*. 2014;33:136-9.

43. Smijs TG, Pavel S. The susceptibility of dermatophytes to photodynamic treatment with special focus on *Trichophyton rubrum. Photochem Photobiol*. 2011;87:2-13.

44. Weber GC, Firouzi P, Baran AM, et al. Treatment of onychomycosis using a 1064-nm diode laser with or without topical antifungal therapy: a single-center, retrospective analysis in 56 patients. *Eur J Med Res*. 2018;23:53.

45. Gupta AK, Simpson F. Newly approved laser systems for onychomycosis. *J Am Podiatr Med Assoc*. 2012;102:428-30.

46. Carney C, Cantrell W, Warner J, Elewski B. Treatment of onychomycosis using a submillisecond 1064-nm neodymium:yttrium-aluminum-garnet laser. *J Am Acad Dermatol*. 2013;69:578-82.

47. Ardeshna KP, Rohatgi S, Jerajani HR. Successful treatment of recurrent dermatophytosis with isotretinoin and itraconazole. *Indian J Dermatol Venereol Leprol*. 2016;82:579-82.

48. Narang T. Isotretinoin in preventing recurrences in chronic recurrent dermatophytosis (ISORD). (2018). [online] Available from https://clinicaltrials.gov/ct2/show/NCT03471455. [Last accessed February, 2019].

49. Lund A, Deboer DJ. Immunoprophylaxis of dermatophytosis in animals. *Mycopathologia*. 2008;166:407-24.

50. Rajagopalan M, Inamadar A, Mittal A, et al. Expert consensus on the management of dermatophytosis in India (ECTODERM India). *BMC Dermatol*. 2018;18(1):6.

World Clin Dermatol. 2019;5(1):29-40.

Other Cutaneous Superficial Fungal Infections and their Topical Treatment

[1],*Nisha V Parmar MD, [2]Rashmi Sarkar MD MNAMS

[1]Department of Dermatology, Rashid Hospital, Dubai Health Authority
Dubai, United Arab Emirates
[2]Department of Dermatology, STD and Leprosy, Maulana Azad Medical College and
Lok Nayak Hospital, New Delhi, India

ABSTRACT

The topical therapy of other superficial fungal infections will be covered in this article. Conditions covered include those commonly encountered in day-to-day practice such as pityriasis versicolor and mucocutaneous candidiasis, as well as the rarer condition tinea nigra.

INTRODUCTION

Pityriasis Versicolor

Pityriasis versicolor (PV) is a common superficial fungal infection caused by the *Malassezia* species. *Malassezia* are dimorphic lipophilic fungi that exist as normal skin flora and become pathogenic under conditions such as a humid environment, increased sebum secretion, familial susceptibility and an immunocompromised state. Under these conditions, the yeast form gets transformed into a pathogenic mycelial form and produces skin lesions in the form of hypopigmented, hyperpigmented, or sometimes, erythematous scaly macules with fine branny scales (Figure 1). The yeasts are abundant in the seborrheic areas of the body due to their lipophilicity, and hence, lesions of PV are seen on the trunk, face and flexures.

*Corresponding author
Email: parmarnish@gmail.com

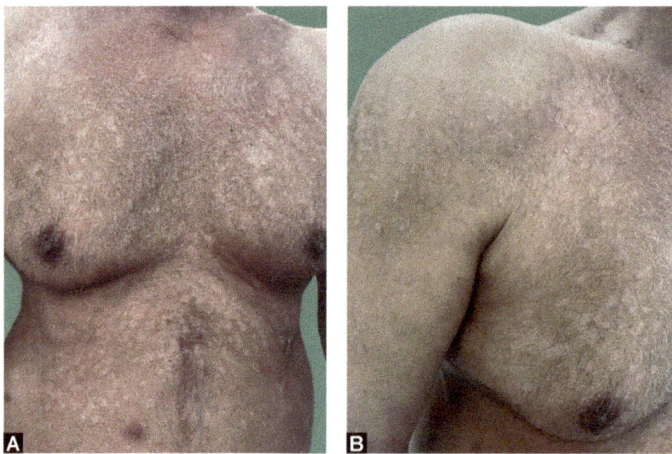

Figure 1: Pityriasis versicolor—hypopigmented and hyperpigmented lesions with branny scaling.

Amongst the 13 *Malassezia* species currently existing, the most common species causing PV are in order as *Malassezia globosa*, *Malassezia sympodialis* and *Malassezia furfur*.[1]

Pityriasis versicolor tends to be chronic and recurrent in susceptible individuals. Recurrence occurs in about 60% of patients at 1 year and 80–90% at 2 years.[2]

Treatment is aimed at providing symptomatic relief albeit temporary. Pigmentation abnormality may take months to heal, hence, does not indicate treatment failure and patients need to be adequately informed.

The first-line treatment of PV is topical antifungals. Oral therapy is indicated in patients with widespread lesions or those who fail topical therapy. Topical therapy is further classified into traditional or nonspecific antifungal agents and specific antifungal treatment.[3]

Nonspecific Topical Antifungal Agents

These agents were the initially utilized treatments for PV. They do not have any direct antifungal activity but act via mechanical removal of the stratum corneum, and hence, secondarily lead to removal of the fungi which are residents of the stratum corneum. Agents in this group include selenium sulfide, zinc pyrithione, Whitfield's ointment and propylene glycol.

Selenium sulfide is available as 2.5% shampoo, lotion, and cream. It is to be applied to the affected areas for 5–10 minutes and washed during shower. Treatment regimens include once daily for 1 week and once a week for 4 weeks.[4]

Zinc pyrithione is available as 1% shampoo which is to be applied to the affected area for 5–10 minutes, then washed off. When applied once daily for 2 weeks, it is found to be an effective treatment of PV.[5]

Whitfield's ointment consists of 3% salicylic acid and 6% benzoic acid. It is a traditional treatment that acts via its keratolytic effect.[3]

All these agents can cause irritation, dryness and transient burning.

Specific Topical Antifungal Agents

These agents include topical azoles, topical allylamine and benzylamine antifungals, all of which are effective against *Malassezia*.

Topical Azole Antifungal Agents for Pityriasis Versicolor

Topical azoles are the first-line treatment for PV. The imidazole subgroup of azole antifungals is particularly effective against PV. Imidazoles include ketoconazole, clotrimazole, miconazole, econazole, oxiconazole, flutrimazole, tioconazole, fenticonazole and bifonazole. These agents act via inhibiting the cytochrome P450-dependant enzyme lanosterol-14-α-demethylase necessary for fungal cell membrane synthesis. Inhibition of this enzyme leads to arrest in fungal cell growth, thus, having a fungistatic effect.

Topical Ketoconazole

Two percent ketoconazole is an age-old treatment which is till date very effective against the *Malassezia* yeasts. It is the most extensively used and studied treatment of PV. It is available as shampoo, cream and more recently foam.

Various regimens of application have been used ranging from single application to once daily application for 14 days. Lange et al. conducted a double-blinded randomized placebo-controlled multicenter trial evaluating the efficacy of single application of 2% ketoconazole shampoo versus once daily application of the same for 3 days. Patients used either single application of ketoconazole shampoo for 5–10 minutes followed by placebo for 2 days, once daily application of ketoconazole for 3 days or placebo alone for 3 days. Both ketoconazole regimens did not show any statistically significant difference in their mycological cure rates (daily application for 3 days had a mycological cure rate of 84% and single application, a cure rate of 78% vs. the 11% cure rate of placebo). The relapse rates with these regimens were found to be higher when patients were followed up for 3–24 months post-treatment.[6]

Two percent ketoconazole foam is the only new antifungal product to be added in the armamentarium for the treatment of PV. It has shown promising results in maintenance of long term remission when used once daily for 14 days. After evaporation, increased trascutaneous penetration allows for the desired concentration to remain in the stratum corneum for longer, hence longer remission rates are seen.[7]

Other Topical Azoles

Clotrimazole, a topical imidazole antifungal is effective in a 1% cream and solution form for the treatment of PV. One percent clotrimazole cream twice daily for 2 weeks was compared to single dose of fluconazole 400 mg. The subjects were evaluated at the end of 2 weeks, then at 4 weeks and 12 weeks. At the end of 2 weeks, there was a statistically significant difference in resolution of lesions in the clotrimazole group compared to the fluconazole group. However, recurrence rate at 12 weeks was higher in the clotrimazole group compared to the fluconazole group (18.2% vs. 6%).[8]

Econazole and miconazole are synthetic imidazole topical antifungals. Econazole as a 1% cream, foam, or shampoo and miconazole as a 2% cream applied once daily for 2 weeks are effective first-line treatments for PV.[9,10]

Sertaconazole is a broad-spectrum antifungal cream available as 1% or 2% concentrations. The treatment duration is longer and twice daily application for 4 weeks is found to be effective for PV.[11]

Bifonazole is available in many formulations. A single application was also found to be effective in treating PV. It is available as 1% cream, foam, spray, powder and gel.[12]

Other imidazole creams which have proved effective in treating PV include tioconazole 1%, fenticonazole 1% and flutrimazole 1%.

Topical Allylamine Antifungals

Topical allyamines include terbinafine and naftifine. This group of agents is fungicidal and acts via inhibition of squalene epoxidase enzyme, hence, leading to accumulation of squalene and subsequent death of the fungus. Topical terbinafine is effective against the *Malassezia* yeasts. Terbinafine is available as 1% cream and 1% solution. Most studies with terbinafine cream have evaluated its use as twice daily for 4 weeks and found equal efficacy as 2% ketoconazole at 88–100%.[13] Terbinafine solution applied twice daily for 7 days produced mycological cure rates of around 81%, 7 weeks after treatment completion.[14-16]

Table 1 represents a summary of double blinded randomized controlled trials investigating the various topical antifungals for PV.

Treatment regimen	No. of subjects	Clinical cure rate	Mycological cure rate	Complete cure	Follow-up, if any
Table 1: A Summary of Randomized Double-blinded Trials of Topical Antifungals for Pityriasis Versicolor*					
Sanchez et al.[4]					
A. Selenium sulfide 2.5% lotion once daily for 1 week	48	NA	39	NA	NA
B. Selenium sulfide 2.5% lotion + 0.2% colorants once daily for 1 week	38	NA	27	NA	NA
C. Vehicle + 0.2% colorants once daily for 1 week	36	NA	7	NA	NA
Savin et al.[17]					
Ketoconazole 2% cream vs. placebo once daily for 11–22 days	51 vs. 50	34 (67%) vs. 11 (22%)	43 (84%) 11 (22%)	43 (84%) 5 (10%)	At 1 year, complete cure rates in treatment group 42/51 (82%) At 2 years, complete cure in treatment group 16/51 (33%)
Balwada et al.[18]					
A. Ketoconazole 2% cream daily for 14 days	20		18/20 (90%)	18/20 (90%)	At 8 weeks 16/16 (100%)
B. Clotrimazole 1% cream	20		17/20 (85%)	16/20 (80%)	16/16 (100%)
Lange et al.[6]					
A. Ketoconazole 2% shampoo once on day 1 then placebo once a day for next 2 days	103				At 31 days Clinical cure 71/103 (69%) Mycological cure 79/103 (78%)
B. Ketoconazole 2% shampoo once daily for 3 days	106				Clinical cure 77/106 (73%) Mycological cure 89/106 (84%)
C. Placebo once daily for 3 days	103				Clinical cure 11 (11%) Mycological cure 5 (5%)

Continued

33

Continued

Table 1: A Summary of Randomized Double-blinded Trials of Topical Antifungals for Pityriasis Versicolor*

Treatment regimen	No. of subjects	Clinical cure rate	Mycological cure rate	Complete cure	Follow-up, if any
Rigopoulos et al.[19]					
A. Ketoconazole 2% shampoo once a day for 14 days	26				At day 28: Mycologic cure 21/26 (81%)
B. Flutrimazole 1% shampoo once a day for 14 days	29				22/29 (76%)
Di Fonzo et al.[7]					
A. Ketoconazole 1% foam once daily for 14 days versus	22				At 5 weeks, 29% complete resolution at 5 weeks At 3 months, 82% complete resolution
B. Ketoconazole 2% cream once daily for 14 days	24				At 5 weeks, 47% complete resolution At 3 months, 92% complete resolution
Shi et al.[20]					
A. Ketoconazole 2% cream + 0.1% adapalene gel once daily for 14 days	50				At 4 weeks, Mycolcogic cure: 46/50 (92%)
B. Ketoconazole 2% cream twice daily for 14 days	50				36/50 (72%)
Vermeer et al.[14]					
Terbinafine 1% solution vs. placebo twice daily for 1 week	76 34	55 (72%) 9 (26%)	At 8 weeks 62 (81%) 14 (41%)	47% vs. 29%	
Savin et al.[15]					
A. Terbinafine 1% solution vs. vehicle twice daily for 7 days	96 46	45 (47%) 14 (30%)	At 1 week 57 (59%) 26 (56%)		At 8 weeks, clinical cure rate 81% vs. 31%, Mycological cure rate 82% vs. 32%

Continued

Continued

| Table 1: A Summary of Randomized Double-blinded Trials of Topical Antifungals for Pityriasis Versicolor* ||||||
Treatment regimen	No. of subjects	Clinical cure rate	Mycological cure rate	Complete cure	Follow-up, if any
Budimulja et al.[16]					
A. Terbinafine 1% solution vs. vehicle twice daily for 1 week	192 vs. 96		At 2 weeks, 108 (56%) vs. 34 (35%) in group		Mycological cure at 8 weeks: 123 (64%) vs. 32 (33%) in group A and 25 (50%) vs. 14 (28%) in group B
B. Terbinafine 1% solution once daily for 1 week	50 vs. 50				
Faergemann et al.[21]					
Terbinafine 1% emulsion gel vs. placebo gel once daily for 1 week	31 vs. 30			11/29 (39%) vs. 7/29 (24%)	At 8 weeks, 21/28 (75%) vs. 4/29 (14%) remained completely cured
Alomar et al.[22]					
Flutrimazole 1% cream vs. bifonazole 1% cream once daily for 4 weeks	228 221			166 (73%) 144 (66%)	
Vicik et al.[9]					
1% econazole nitrate vs. placebo once daily for 2–3 weeks	67 vs. 59		At 3 weeks, 53 (79%) vs. 37 (63%)		
Spiekermann et al.[23]					
A. Clotrimazole 1% solution vs. vehicle once daily for 2 weeks	116 vs. 107	96 (83%) vs. 68 (64%)	96 (83%) vs. 68 (64%)		
B. Clotrimazole 1% cream once daily for 2 weeks	10 vs. 8	8 (80) vs. 3 (38%)	8 (80) vs. 3 (38%)		

*Only studies with more than 20 patients in each group are presented here.

Topical Antifungal Prophylactic Therapy for Pityriasis Versicolor

The recurrence rates of PV tend to be very high, approaching 60–90% at 2 years. Few topical regimens have been recommended for prophylaxis:

- Application of ketoconazole shampoo for 5–10 minutes followed by shower for 3 days at the beginning of summer is advocated to prevent recurrences[24]
- Application of ketoconazole, selenium sulfide or zinc pyrithione shampoo for 5–10 minutes 1–4 times a month.[25]

TINEA NIGRA

Tinea nigra is a superficial fungal infection caused by the dematiaceous fungus *Hortaea werneckii*. It presents as sharply demarcated brown to black macules with irregular edges commonly on the palms and soles after an incubation period of 10–15 days. It is diagnosed by demonstration of the pigmented fungal hyphae on potassium hydroxide mount.

Treatment

Tinea nigra responds excellently to the azole antifungals as well as allylamines and benzylamine. Topical antifungals that have been found to successfully cure the condition include ketoconazole, isoconazole, bifonazole, butenafine, terbinafine usually within 2–4 weeks.[26] Response is also seen with keratolytic agents such as Whitfield's ointment alone or in combination with topical antifungals.

MUCOCUTANEOUS CANDIDIASIS

Candidiasis is a superficial fungal infection of the skin and mucous membranes caused by yeasts of the genus *Candida*. *Candida albicans* is the most common and well known member of this genus. Other clinically significant *Candida* species include *C. glabrata*, *C. dubliniensis*, *C. parapsilosis*, *C. tropicalis*, *C. pseudotropicalis* and *C. guilliermondii*. Whereas *C. albicans* was traditionally the most frequent isolated from various infections, the scenario is gradually changing with one or more of the above species being the most common in a few countries.

Candidiasis is a regular opportunistic infection in states of lowered systemic and cutaneous immunity such as diabetes, human immunodeficiency virus (HIV) infection, in patients receiving systemic and topical steroids. It also occurs due to suppression of local bacterial flora and ph in those receiving systemic antibiotics.

Management of Candidiasis at Different Cutaneous Sites

The first-line treatment of mucocutaneous candidiasis is topical antifungals. The agents effective against *Candida* include:

- Polyene antifungals—amphotericin B and nystatin
- Imidazole antifungals—clotrimazole, miconazole, econazole
- Allylamines—terbinafine, naftifine, and benzylamine butenafine.

Unfortunately, most of the studies for candidiasis focus on esophageal and vaginal candidiasis, hence, trials for treatment of cutaneous candidiasis are lacking.

General Principles

In general, certain principles of care have to be taken into account when treating mucocutaneous candidiasis:

- For cutaneous infections, keeping the affected area dry is of prime importance. In case of bedridden patients for example, periodic change in position is advised to prevent continuous occlusion and moisture retention which favor growth of *Candida*
- For oral candidiasis frequent cleansing and care of dentures, when used, are to be emphasized upon.

Oral Candidiasis

Oral candidiasis is seen commonly in newborns and infants. In adults, denture use, diabetes, oral antibiotic use, and HIV infection are all predisposing factors. The diagnosis is usually confirmed by a potassium hydroxide mount.

For treating oral thrush in infants, nystatin suspension, clotrimazole oral paint, miconazole oral gel, and amphotericin gel (where available) are effective and adequate when applied several times a day.

In immunocompetent adults, general care measures like frequent mouth washes and care of dentures at night should be counseled. Topical therapy in the form of clotrimazole oral paint, miconazole oral gel, nystatin oral suspension and amphotericin or nystatin lozenges are sufficient in addition to general care measures.[27]

In the immunocompromised patient, topical antifungals are often ineffective and systemic antifungal therapy is required.

Genital Candidiasis

Vulvovaginal candidiasis (VVC) affects 75% of women of child-bearing age. Its manifestations include curdy white discharge per vaginum, soreness, itching and a macerated appearance of the vulva. It can be recurrent in 5% of patients.[28] First-line treatment includes oral antifungals, and fluconazole 150 mg as a single dose is the standard treatment. Itraconazole 600 mg single dose is an alternative. Topical antifungals play a role in management of vulvar erythema and maceration: clotrimazole, miconazole and econazole creams applied twice daily for 2 weeks are effective for this.

Mild cases of candidal balanitis and balanoposthitis present with asymptomatic pustules which may rupture to leave fine scale after sexual contact with an infected partner and may heal spontaneously or progress to frank maceration. Uncontrolled diabetes is also a predisposing factor. Treatment of all patients with candidal balanitis or balanoposthitis is with topical antifungals alone with applications of clotrimazole, miconazole or econazole creams several times a day.[28] Where the partner is the source of infection, she should also be treated as above mentioned.

Candidal Intertrigo

Candidiasis of the folds can affect any fold of the body and is more common in obese individuals. Topical steroids prescribed for relief of symptoms only aggravate the situation by allowing multiplication of the fungus. The general measures have to be advised and the affected areas should be kept dry. Open shoes should be worn by those with interdigital candidiasis.

The mainstay of treatment are topical polyene and imidazole antifungal creams applied twice daily for 2 weeks.

Napkin Candidiasis

In infants, *Candida* is a common isolate of the skin of the buttocks. However, if there is an underlying diaper rash, candidiasis can be a superimposed infection especially if there is use of an antibacterial cream with subsequent suppression of the bacterial flora.[29]

The presence of redness, maceration, satellite papules and pustules points toward a diagnosis of candidiasis. Once this is confirmed the following should be done:

Frequent change of diapers is advocated. Avoidance of topical steroids and use of an antifungal cream such as clotrimazole, miconazole and econazole several times a day for 1–2 weeks is sufficient.

Candidiasis of the Nail and Paronychium

Candida species can also affect the nail and paronychium. Predisposing factors include diabetes with associated poor peripheral circulation and continuous wet work. Repeated assault to the paronychium results in its separation from the nail plate, leading to pocketing. The pockets may harbor thick pus when expressed. With chronic insult, nail dystrophy may occur in the affected nail.[30]

Management includes control of diabetes in those with it, avoidance of and precautions with wet work, and topical antifungals. Lotions and solutions are preferred to creams.

First-line treatments include topical azole antifungal solution twice daily for 2–4 months. In addition, in chronic cases, a medium potency topical steroid cream has to be applied once daily.

CONCLUSION

Topical azole antifungals are the first-line therapy for treatment of PV and mucocutaneous candidiasis. For mucocutaneous candidiasis, general measures play a key role in management and should be emphasized upon. For tinea nigra, topical treatment is sufficient and allylamines, azoles and keratolytic agents all work excellently.

REFERENCES

1. Gupta AK, Kohli Y, Summerbell RC, Faergemann J. Quantitative culture of Malassezia species from different body sites of individuals with or without dermatoses. *Med Mycol.* 2001;39(3):243-51.
2. Faergemann J. The role of *Malassezia* yeasts in skin diseases. *Mikol Lek.* 2004;11:129-33.
3. Gupta AK, Kogan N, Batra R. Pityriasis versicolor: a review of pharmacology treatment options. *Expert Opin Pharmacother.* 2005;6(2):165-78.
4. Sánchez JL, Torres VM. Double-blind efficacy study of selenium sulfide in tinea versicolor. *J Am Acad Dermatol.* 1984;11(2 Pt 1):235-8.
5. Faergemann J, Fredriksson T. An open trial of the effect of a zinc pyrithione shampoo in tinea versicolor. *Cutis.* 1980;25(6):667,669.
6. Lange DS, Richards HM, Guarnieri J, et al. Ketoconazole 2% shampoo in the treatment of tinea versicolor: a multicenter, randomized, double-blind, placebo-controlled trial. *J Am Acad Dermatol.* 1998;39(6):944-50.
7. Di Fonzo EM, Martini P, Mazzatenta C, Lotti L, Alvino S. Comparative efficacy and tolerability of ketomaousse (ketoconazole foam 1%) and ketoconazole cream 2% in the treatment of pityriasis versicolor: Results of a prospective, multicenter, randomized study. *Mycoses.* 2008;51(6):532-5.
8. Dehghan M, Akbari N, Alborzi N, Sadani S, Keshtkar AA. Single-dose oral fluconazole versus topical clotrimazole in patients with pityriasis versicolor: a double-blind randomized control trial. *J Dermatol.* 2010;37(8):699-702.
9. Vicik GJ, Mendiones M, Quinones CA, Thorne EG. A new treatment for tinea versicolor using econazole nitrate 1.0 percent cream once a day. *Cutis.* 1984;33(6)570-1.

10. Tanenbaum L, Anderson C, Rosenberg MJ, Akers W. 1% sulconazole cream v 2% miconazole cream in the treatment of tinea versicolor. A double-blind, multicenter study. *Arch Dermatol.* 1984;120(2):216-9.

11. Nassare J, Umbert P, Herrero E, et al. Therapeutic efficacy and safety of the new antimycotic sertaconazole in the treatment of pityriasis versicolor. *Arzneimittelforschung.* 1992;42(5A):764-7.

12. Mora RG, Greer DL. Comparative efficacy and tolerance of 1% bifonazole cream and bifonazole cream vehicle in patients with tinea versicolor. *Dermatologica.* 1984;169(Suppl 1):87-92.

13. Chopra V, Jain VK. Comparative study of topical terbinafine and topical ketoconazole in pityriasis versicolor. *Indian J Dermatol Venereol Leprol.* 2000;66(6):299-300.

14. Vermeer BJ, Staats CC. The efficacy of a topical application of terbinafine 1% solution in subjects with pityriasis versicolor: a placebo-controlled study. *Dermatology.* 1997;194(Suppl 1):22-4.

15. Savin R, Eisen D, Fradin MS, Lebwohl M. Tinea versicolor treated with terbinafine 1% solution. *Int J Dermatol.* 1999;31(11):863-5.

16. Budimulja U, Paul C. One-week terbinafine 1% solution in pityriasis versicolor: twice-daily application is more effective than once-daily. *J Dermatolog Treat.* 2002;13(1):39-40

17. Savin RC, Horwitz SN. Double-blind comparison of 2% ketoconazole cream and placebo in the treatment of tinea versicolor. *J Am Acad Dermatol.* 1986;15(3):500-3.

18. Balwada RP, Jain VK, Dayal S. A double-blind comparison of 2% ketoconazole and 1% clotrimazole in the treatment of pityriasis versicolor. *Indian J Dermatol Venereol Leprol.* 1996;62(5):298-300.

19. Rigopoulos D, Gregoriou S, Kontochristopoulos G, Ifantides A, Katsambas A. Flutrimazole shampoo 1% versus ketoconazole shampoo 2% in the treatment of pityriasis versicolor. A randomised double-blind comparative trial. *Mycoses.* 2007;50(3):193-5.

20. Shi TW, Zhang JA, Tang YB, et al. A randomized controlled trial of combination treatment with ketoconazole 2% cream and adapalene 0.1% gel in pityriasis versicolor. *J Dermatolog Treat.* 2015;26(2):143-6.

21. Faergemann J, Hersle K, Nordin P. Pityriasis versicolor: clinical experience with Lamisil cream and Lamisil DermGel. *Dermatology.* 1997;194(Suppl 1):19-21.

22. Alomar S, Videla S, Delgadillo J, et al. Flutrimazole 1% dermal cream in the treatment of dermatomycoses: a multicenter, double-blind, randomized, comparative clinical trial with bifonazole 1% cream. Efficacy of flutrimazole 1% dermal cream in dermatomycoses. Catalan Flutrimazole study Group. *Dermatology.* 1995;190(4):295-300.

23. Spiekermann PH, Young MD. Clinical evaluation of clotrimazole. A broad-spectrum antifungal agent. *Arch Dermatol.* 1976;112(3):350-2.

24. Hu SW, Bigby M. Pityriasis versicolor: a systematic review of interventions. *Arch Dermatol.* 2010;146(10): 1132-40.

25. Renati S, Cukras A, Bigby M. Pityriasis versicolor. *BMJ.* 2015;350:h1394.

26. Bonifaz A, Gómez-Daza F, Paredes V, Ponce RM. Tinea versicolor, tinea nigra, white piedra, and black piedra. *Clin Dermatol.* 2010;28(2):140-5.

27. Dreizen S. Oral candidiasis. *Am J Med.* 1984;77(4D):28-33.

28. Odds FC. Genital candidosis. *Clin Exp Dermatol.* 1982;7:343-54.

29. Šikić Pogacar M, Maver U, Marčun Varda N, Mičetić-Turk D. Diagnosis and management of diaper dermatitis in infants with emphasis on skin microbiota in the diaper area. *Int J Dermatol.* 2018;57(3):265-75.

30. Hay RJ, Baran R, Moore MK, Wilkinson JD. Candida onychomycosis—an evaluation of the role of Candida species in nail disease. *Br J Dermatol.* 1988;118(1):47-58.

World Clin Dermatol. 2019;5(1):41-56.

Onychomycoses—Latest Developments and Topical Treatment

[1]Somodyuti Chandra MD DNB SCE (UK), [2,*]Indrashis Podder MD DNB

[1]Venkat Center for Skin and Plastic Surgery
Bengaluru, Karnataka, India
[2]Department of Dermatology, College of Medicine and Sagore Dutta Hospital
Kolkata, West Bengal, India

ABSTRACT

Onychomycosis refers to fungal infection of the nail unit including the nail plate, nail bed and the periungual tissue, accounting for almost half of all nail disorders. *Trichophyton rubrum* and *Trichophyton mentagrophytes* are the most common causative organisms. Topical treatment is a very important part of therapy, with newer drugs evolving at a rapid pace. However, long-term treatment is needed to achieve both clinical and mycological cure, thus escalating the cost burden and chance of adverse effects. So, several natural remedies are being considered as adjunctive measures to counter these adversities.

INTRODUCTION

Onychomycosis is a fungal infection of the nail unit, involving the nail plate, nail bed and the periungual tissue. It has a worldwide prevalence of 5.5% and represents about 50% of all nail disorders seen in dermatology practice.[1] It is characterized by thickening, discoloration, splitting of nail plate and its separation from the nail bed, this disorder is more than mere cosmetic distress or social embarrassment. Though generally not life-threatening, untreated infections can cause pain, discomfort and difficulty in mobility and may even progress to other parts of the nail unit, including the nail matrix, causing destruction and deformity of the finger- and toenails. Onychomycosis, especially those caused by dermatophytes,

---

*Corresponding author
Email: ipodder@gmail.com

serve as a nidus of infection and can spread to other digits, body areas or even other susceptible contacts.

The majority of cases of onychomycosis are caused by dermatophyte fungi, commonly *Trichophyton rubrum* and *Trichophyton mentagrophytes*. Other organisms like yeast (such as *Candida* species) and nondermatophyte molds (such as *Fusarium* species, *Acremonium* species, *Aspergillus* species, *Scytalidium* species and *Scopulariopsis* species) account for about 10% of nail infections globally[2] and mixed infections too are not uncommon.

The United States Food and Drug Administration (USFDA) has set down certain treatment efficacy endpoints in relation to onychomycosis clinical trials that are based on physical examination, fungal culture and microscopy. The primary endpoint recognized by the USFDA is complete cure while the secondary endpoints are clinical cure and mycological cure. Mycological cure is defined as negative potassium hydroxide (KOH) microscopy and no growth in culture, while clinical cure is defined as completely normal appearing nails. Complete cure is essentially a combination of both, i.e. elimination of fungal elements coupled with the formation of new, clear, intact nail plate. However, sometimes long-standing infection can permanently damage the nail matrix or nail bed leading to dystrophic and discolored nails despite mycological cure.

HISTORY

Over the years, treatment of onychomycosis has evolved greatly. Till 1938, potassium permanganate ($KMnO_4$) soaks, Castellani's carbol-fuchsin paint and sandpaper were the mainstay of therapy while formaldehyde vapor was used to disinfect shoes and gloves. In 1958, griseofulvin became the first oral drug to be approved by USFDA for the treatment of onychomycosis which in 1981 was superseded by oral ketoconazole owing to its better efficacy and shorter treatment course. Later, as ketoconazole use began to decline because of severe hepatic side effects, itraconazole and terbinafine were granted USFDA approval in 1995 and 1996, respectively.[3] In 1999, ciclopirox was the first topical drug to be approved for onychomycosis. More than a decade later, in 2014, two new topicals efinaconazole and tavaborole were added to the armamentarium.

TOPICAL TREATMENT

As the occurrence levels of onychomycosis keep on increasing nowadays, need of topical therapy that can circumvent the threats posed by systemic delivery is gaining prominent deliberations. Generally used along with oral drugs, specific indications for their monotherapy have not been clearly elucidated. However, it is useful in treating infections with limited nail involvement, such as distal-lateral onychomycosis involving less than 50% of nail plate without nail matrix involvement; infections without substantial nail plate thickening, i.e. nail thickness should be less than 2 mm; superficial white type of onychomycosis and in presence of few three or four affected nails.[4]

Topical therapy has several advantages over oral antifungal therapy. Acting locally at the target site, there is minimal plasma accumulation of the drug, and thus are devoid of systemic side effects and drug-drug interactions; do not need laboratory monitoring and can be used unhindered in presence of comorbid conditions, such as hepatic or renal dysfunction while achieving a cure rate comparable to the systemic drugs.

Despite possessing attractive benefits, topical therapy is met with various challenges like suboptimal vehicles delivering the drug to its site of action, poor penetration of drug molecules through the keratinized nail plate into the nail bed and achievement of inadequate therapeutic concentration in the nail bed. The drug must be of small size, hydrophilic, nonionic and sublimable to attain desired concentration in the deeper layers of the nail.[5] In addition, certain clinical patterns of involvement make the scenario even more challenging; as in cases of extensive nail plate involvement along with profound matrix damage, presence of onycholysis, marked nail plate thickening, gross subungual hyperkeratosis, band-like lateral involvement and presence of dermatophytoma (i.e. formation of fungal ball containing numerous fungal elements admixed in fungal spores, bound together by biofilm).[6] Owing to the slow growth rate of nails, adherence to therapy for more than 6 months for fingernail (having growth rate 2–3 mm/month) (Figure 1) and 12–18 months for toenail (having growth rate 1–2 mm/month) infection is an important determinant affecting fungal clearance and chance of recurrence.

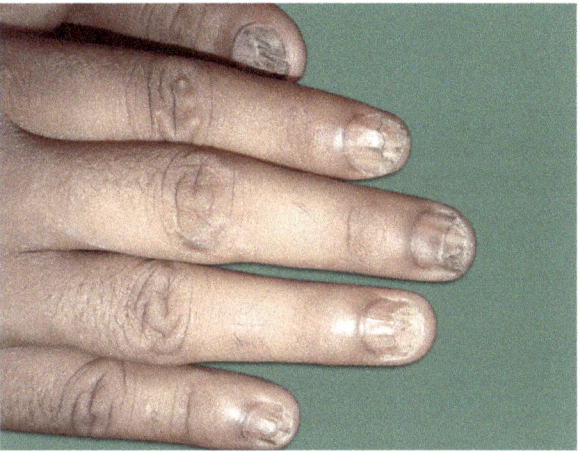

Figure 1: Onychomycosis of all fingernails.

Table 1: Topical Agents for Treatment of Onychomycosis	
Pharmacologic agents/drugs	**Nonpharmacologic/over-the-counter natural remedies**
<ul><li>USFDA-approved<ul><li>Ciclopirox olamine 8% nail lacquer*</li><li>Efinaconazole 10% solution</li><li>Tavaborole 5% solution</li></ul></li><li>Non-USFDA approved<ul><li>Amorolfine 5% nail lacquer*</li></ul></li><li>Newer investigational drugs<ul><li>Terbinafine nail solution</li><li>Luliconazole 10% solution</li></ul></li></ul>	<ul><li>Tea tree oil</li><li>Natural topical cough suppressants</li><li>Natural coniferous nail lacquer</li><li>*Ageratina pichinchensis* extract</li><li>Ozonized sunflower oil</li></ul>

*Patients must file and trim nails weekly.

Topical formulations for onychomycosis are available in the form of creams, solutions and lacquers. While topical solutions and creams can be readily removed by wiping or washing, nail lacquers being volatile, evaporate leaving a clear, stable, occlusive film on the nail surface. This film acts as a drug depot, releasing the active drug for a specified period of time. Also, the film prevents tranonychial water loss, hydrates the keratin layers of the nail plate and further facilitates transungual penetration of drug moiety.[7] Apart from pharmacologic medications/drugs, several nonpharmacologic, over-the-counter, natural remedies have shown variable antifungal actions in in vitro studies.[8] However, their widespread use is not yet recommended due to lack of large scale clinical trials.

The different topical agents which are being considered for treatment of onychomycosis have been tabulated in Table 1.

Ciclopirox

Ciclopirox nail lacquer was the first topical antifungal to be approved by the USFDA in December 1999 for mild-to-moderate onychomycosis of finger- and toenail in immunocompetent patients. This synthetic broad-spectrum antifungal has additional antibacterial, anti-inflammatory and antiallergic properties. It is a pregnancy category B drug.

Structure

It is a member of the hydroxypyridone [6-cyclohexyl-1-hydroxy-4-methyl-2(1H)-pyridone] family and the hydroxyl group is vital for its antimicrobial effect.[9]

Mechanism of Action

Ciclopirox acts by interfering with the metabolic activity in the fungal cell. It chelates polyvalent cations like Fe^{3+} and Al^{3+} that are essential cofactors of cytochromal enzymes and inactivates fungal catalases and peroxidases. Consequently, intracellular energy production is hampered along with accumulation of toxic peroxides leading to oxidative damage to the cell. Additionally, it is also found to inhibit nutrient uptake by the fungal cell, thereby depleting amino acids and nucleotides and impairing protein and nucleic acid synthesis.[9]

Its anti-inflammatory effect is exerted by inhibition of formation and release of inflammatory mediators (like prostaglandins) and scavenging reactive oxygen species released from the inflammatory cells.[10]

Antimicrobial Spectrum of Activity

Ciclopirox is fungicidal against all dermatophytes (*Trichophyton* species, *Epidermophyton* species and *Microsporum* species), *Candida* species as well as nondermatophyte molds, particularly *Scytalidium hyalinum* which is resistant to most antifungals. It has also shown to be effective against gram-positive and gram-negative bacteria, both aerobes and anaerobes. Onychomycosis is frequently complicated by secondary bacterial infection and ciclopirox is highly beneficial in such instances.[9-10]

Pharmacokinetic Properties

In vitro experiments using radiolabeled ciclopirox showed that after 24 hours of single application on an avulsed toenail, the drug penetrated the full thickness of the nail plate measuring about 80–120 μm and attained a concentration of 29 μg/g in the innermost layer which is much higher than the minimum inhibitory concentration (MIC) of less than 4 μg/mL for most causative organisms.[9] Moreover, the degree of penetration was found to be enhanced in the diseased nails having structural changes like rough, fissured nail plate. After 7–14 days of application, biologically effective concentration of ciclopirox can be attained at all layers of the nail and persists up to 14 days of termination of therapy.

Clinical Effects

Mycological cure and complete cure rates (Figures 2 and 3) with ciclopirox are found to be 29–36% and 5.5–8.5% respectively compared to placebo, which has a complete cure rate of 0–0.9%.[11]

45

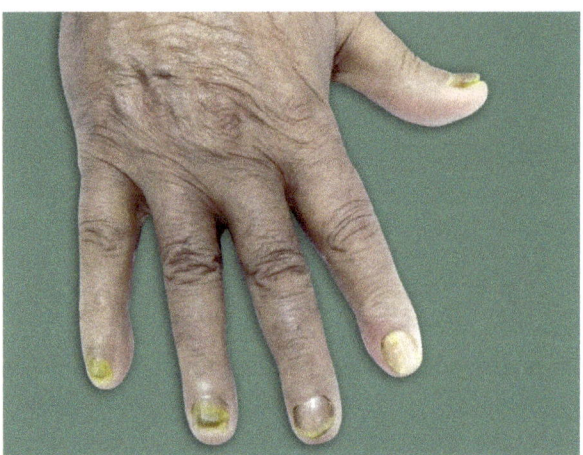

Figure 2: Baseline picture showing onychomycosis.

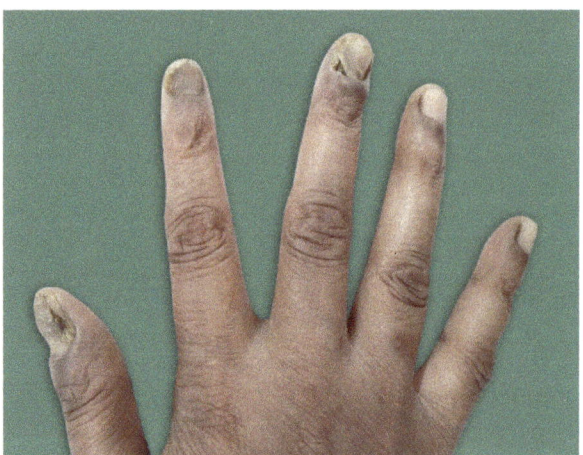

Figure 3: Post-treatment picture showing considerable improvement.

Dosage and Administration

Ciclopirox 8% nail lacquer is to be applied daily to the affected nail plate and 5 mm of the surrounding skin for up to 24 weeks for fingernail and 48 weeks for toenail. Washing of the nails should be avoided for about 6–8 hours. After 7 days of continuous use, the lacquer should be removed with alcohol and the nails trimmed and filed to reduce nail thickness for the ease of drug penetration.

Adverse Effects

Ciclopirox nail lacquers are usually well tolerated. The most common adverse events reported include mild inflammatory reaction (i.e. erythema of proximal and lateral nail folds), tingling and burning sensation at the application site. Infrequent side effects noted with ciclopirox as well as the isolated vehicle include change in nail shape, discoloration and onychocryptosis. However, these effects are usually mild and disappear with continuous use.[11]

Amorolfine

Amorolfine, a broad-spectrum antifungal, was introduced in 1981 and is available in Europe and other countries for the treatment of onychomycosis, but not approved in the United States for this indication.

Structure

It is a structurally unique morpholine derivative—4-{3-[p-(1,1-dimethylpropyl)-phenyl]-2-methylpropyl}-2,6-cis-dimethylmorpholine hydrochloride.[12]

Mechanism of Action

Amorolfine, a fungistatic as well as a fungicidal antifungal, acts by interfering with ergosterol biosynthesis by inhibiting two enzymes: (1) delta 14 reductase and (2) delta 7-8 isomerase. Although the effect on these enzymes are both time and concentration dependent, amorolfine exhibits higher affinity for isomerase than reductase enzyme. Consequently, ergosterol is depleted from the fungal cell membrane and instead there is accumulation of ignosterol in *Candida species* and squalene in *Trichophyton species*.[12] These sterols lack the steric configuration required for maintaining the membrane, leading to alteration in the membrane permeability and subsequently the metabolic processes.

Electron microscopic studies have revealed amorolfine additionally damages the cell organelles like mitochondria, nuclei, cytoplasm, cell membrane and cell wall of both *Candida species* and *Trichophyton species*, leading to growth inhibition and ultimately cell death. It does not affect the respiratory transport chain or ribonucleic acid (RNA), deoxyribonucleic acid (DNA), carbohydrate or protein synthesis.[12]

Antimicrobial Spectrum of Activity

Amorolfine has a broad-spectrum of activity against all dermatophyte fungi (*Trichophyton* species, *Epidermophyton* species and *Microsporum* species), pathogenic *Candida* species as well as nondermatophyte molds (*Aspergillus*, *Scytalidium*,

Scopulariopsis), dimorphic fungi and dematiaceous fungi, but has no effect on bacteria except *Actinomyces*. Its fungicidal activity is highest against *T. mentagrophytes*.[13]

Pharmacokinetic Properties

Amorolfine at a concentration of 5% is found to have maximal penetration and therapeutic efficacy. Its penetration profile follows an exponential curve, and the concentration attained in the topmost nail layer is about 100 times that in the lowermost layer.[12]

When 5% amorolfine lacquer is applied, the solvent evaporates leaving a film with the final drug concentration of 25%. The high concentration thus achieved enhances the transungual diffusion of the active drug.

In vitro experiments using radiolabeled amorolfine (3H-labeled 5% amorolfine) in methylene chloride and ethanol lacquers showed that after 48 hours of application, amorolfine attained a concentration of 2.9 µg/mg and 1.2 µg/mg of nail respectively which exceeds the MIC of most fungus causing onychomycosis.[14] It penetrates the nail plate at a rate of 20–100 ng/cm^2/h, reaching a peak at 10–20 hours and subsequently declines slowly, the amount of penetration inversely related to the thickness of the nail plate.[14] Therapeutic efficacy persists for about 14 days after termination of therapy.

Clinical Effects

Mycological cure and complete cure rates with amorolfine are found to be 60–71% and 38–54%, respectively.[3]

Dosage and Administration

Amorolfine 5% nail lacquer should be applied once or twice weekly for a period of 6 months for fingernails and 9–12 months for toenails. Twice weekly application is found to produce higher cure rate; however, it offers no statistically significant benefit compared to once weekly dosing. It is to be applied on the cleaned and filed nails and left to dry for 3–5 minutes. Nail cosmetics including nail polish should not be used on the treated nails.[13]

Amorolfine nail lacquer used every fortnightly for a long time, is effective in preventing recurrent onychomycosis after treatment with oral antifungal.[15]

Adverse Effects

Amorolfine nail lacquer is safe and tolerable. Mild adverse effects reported include inflammatory reaction at the site of application like redness, pain, burning and itching. Concentration of amorolfine and frequency of administration does not influence the frequency of occurrence or the severity of side effects. Systemic absorption is negligible.[13]

Efinaconazole

Efinaconazole, a broad-spectrum triazole, was approved for the treatment of toenail onychomycosis caused by *T. rubrum* and *T. mentagrophytes* in October 2013 in Canada and in June 2014 in the United States. It is a pregnancy category C drug and is contraindicated in pregnancy because of the reported embryotoxic effects on rats. Studies have detected efinaconazole in the breast milk of rats treated with multiple subcutaneous injections, and therefore caution is warranted while prescribing to nursing mothers.[16]

Structure

Previously called IDP-108 and KP-103, efinaconazole was synthesized as an azole amine derivative having the structure 1-piperidineethanol, and α-(2,4-difluorophenyl)-β-methyl-4-methylene-α-(1H-1,2,4-triazol-1-ylmethyl)-, αR, βR-, or (2R,3R)-2-(2,4-difluorophenyl)-3-(4-methylenepiperidin-1-yl)-1-(1H-1,2,4-triazol-1-yl)butan-2-ol.[16]

Mechanism of Action

Efinaconazole acts by interfering with ergosterol biosynthesis by inhibiting the enzyme 4α-demethylase. Loss of ergosterol impairs the fungal cell membrane integrity and ultimately causes cell degeneration and death.

Antimicrobial Spectrum of Activity

Efinaconazole has potent activity against all dermatophyte fungi (*Trichophyton* species, *Epidermophyton* species and *Microsporum* species) particularly *T. rubrum* and *T. mentagrophytes*, pathogenic *Candida* species, *Malassezia furfur*, *Cryptococcus*, *Aspergillus* and other nondermatophyte molds.

Pharmacokinetic Properties

Affinity to keratin is an important property determining penetration and thus availability of optimum concentration of the drug in the deeper layers of the nail.[17] The methylene piperidine group at the C-4 position confers low keratin-binding ability to efinaconazole, contributing to sevenfold higher and faster release rate with better clinical cure with efinaconazole compared to amorolfine, ciclopirox and terbinafine.[17]

In vivo experiments reveal that efinaconazole is absorbed slowly, lacks an elimination phase and metabolized by both oxidation and reduction into a H3 metabolite. Its concentration steadily increases in the nail unit with successive applications reaching MIC values four-fold that for dermatophyte, nondermatophyte and yeast; and the effective levels persist for about 2 weeks after discontinuation of treatment.

It has very low systemic absorption and high affinity for plasma proteins, making the potential for drug-drug interaction almost negligible.[18]

Clinical Effects

Mycological cure and complete cure rates with efinaconazole are 55.2–53.4% and 15.2–17.8%, respectively.[3]

Drug resistance is one of the important causes of treatment failure in onychomycosis as the drugs are typically given for a long time, sometimes over a year. The fungi have been shown to develop drug efflux pumps as a "stress reaction". Both in vitro and in vivo experiments did not show any resistance to efinaconazole.[19]

Dosage and Administration

Efinaconazole 10% solution should be applied once daily for 48 weeks, using a brush applicator provided with the pack. The solution should be applied to all parts of the affected nail, i.e. the nail plate, undersurface of the nail, nail bed, nail folds and hyponychium, ensuring both transungual and subungual delivery of the drug. Commercially available as 4 mL and 8 mL bottles, two drops are required for great toenail and 1 mL for the other toenails. In contrast to the nail lacquers, it does not require removal of the solution or nail filing prior to application. Concomitant use of nail polish should be avoided as it degrades the polish.[18]

Adverse Effects

The most common adverse effects include local application site erythema, pain, blistering, dermatitis and ingrown toenail.[16]

Tavaborole

Tavaborole, previously called AN2690, is the first antifungal of the oxaborole family. It is a unique boron-based molecule that was synthesized from a previous class of boronic acid quinolone compound.[20] It was approved by the USFDA in July 2014 for mild to moderate toenail onychomycosis caused by *T. rubrum* and *T. mentagrophytes*. It is a pregnancy category C drug. Since reduced fetal body weight has been noted in rabbits after topical exposure and its elimination in breast milk is unknown, it is better avoided in pregnancy and lactation.[3]

Structure

Tavaborole ($C_7H_6BFO_2$) has a molecular structure of 1-hydroxy-5-fluoro-1,3-dihydro-2,1-benzoxaborole. The 5-fluoro group and the 1-hydroxyl group provide the compound its unique broad-spectrum antifungal property and hydrophilicity respectively.[20]

Mechanism of Action

Tavaborole has a novel mechanism of action. It inhibits fungal protein synthesis by forming a boron-based bond with the enzyme-editing site of cytoplasmic leucyl-tRNA synthetase. It forms covalent adducts with the tRNA for leucine and blocks the enzyme in the inactive state, interrupting protein synthesis. The affinity to the fungal enzyme is 1,000 times more than the human enzyme, thus imparting specificity.[20]

Antimicrobial Spectrum of Activity

It has a broad-spectrum of activity against *T. rubrum, T. mentagrophytes*, pathogenic *Candida* species, nondermatophyte molds.

Pharmacokinetic Properties

The low keratin-binding property, low-molecular weight (151.93 Da) and volume of the drug, slight water solubility and low surface tension of the vehicle enhance the penetration of tavaborole through the nail plate. It has very low systemic absorption. It is extensively metabolized in the body and excreted via urine. Its concentration in the nail gradually increases with repeated application and the drug can be detected at a concentration more than 17 times the MIC of *T. rubrum* even after 3 months of discontinuation.

Clinical Effects

The mycological and complete cure rates with tavaborole are 31.1–35.9% and 6.5–9.1%, respectively.[21]

Dosage and Administration

Tavaborole 5% solution should be applied once daily for 48 weeks[3] with a pointed-tip glass dropper to the entire nail plate and undersurface of the nail. Removal of previously applied solution and filing is not needed, and it also can be applied in presence of nail polish.

Adverse Effects

The drug is usually well tolerated and has a very low incidence (0.8–2.9%) of mild-to-moderate adverse events that have been reported, which include mainly application site reactions like dermatitis, exfoliation and erythema.[21] These reactions are transient and do not warrant discontinuation of the drug. Systemic absorption of tavaborole is negligible. Animal studies to evaluate genotoxic and carcinogenic potential have also established its safety data.[20]

Newer Topical Drugs under Trial

Apart from the established topical drugs mentioned above, two agents deserve special mention as they are under trial for this purpose:
1. *Terbinafine nail solution*: Phase III clinical trials did not show any added advantage over vehicle/placebo or amorolfine 5% nail lacquer. Headaches, nasopharyngitis and influenza were the most common side effects[3]
2. *10% luliconazole solution*: Luliconazole 1% cream has been recently approved by the USFDA for treatment superficial dermatophytoses caused by *T. rubrum* and *Epidermophyton floccosum*. Recently, a randomized, double-blind phase II/III trial is being conducted to assess the efficacy and safety of 10% luliconazole solution for the treatment of mild-to-moderate onychomycosis.

Nonpharmacologic/Over-the-Counter Natural Remedies

Recently, there has been a renewed interest in natural, over-the-counter, topical nonpharmacologic agents as alternatives to the various medications as they are more cost-effective and have minimal adverse effects. Several authors have demonstrated their efficacy in in vitro laboratory studies; however, their clinical efficacy is doubtful due to lack of large scale clinical trials.[8] These agents may be used as adjuncts to the approved therapeutic options to obtain best results and minimize the occurrence of adverse effects. Some of the important over-the-counter natural remedies are briefly discussed here.

Tea Tree Oil

Tea tree oil (TTO) is a volatile oil extracted from the dried leaves of the *Melaleuca alternifolia* plant, shown to be effective in the treatment of superficial wounds and tinea pedis. Recently, this agent has shown efficacy in the treatment of onychomycosis in both in vitro and clinical trials.

In vitro studies have demonstrated the efficacy of this agent against several fungi including *Candida albicans, T. rubrum, T. mentagrophytes and Aspergillus niger.*[22] Recently, this agent showed considerable efficacy against *T. rubrum* inoculated nail shavings. A nanocapsule and nanoemulsion form has been recently tested and found to be superior to the conventional preparation owing to better penetrability and increased bioavailability.

Two clinical trials have shown therapeutic efficacy of this agent in onychomycosis. Buck et al.[23] showed similar efficacy as clotrimazole 1% solution while Syed et al.[24] demonstrated modest results when used along with another topical antifungal, butenafine hydrochloride 2% cream. In both these studies, TTO was applied twice daily to the affected nails for 8 weeks.

Topical Cough Suppressants

Topical cough suppressants (TCSs) contain several natural ingredients like camphor 4.8%, eucalyptus oil 1.2% and menthol 2.6% (active ingredients) and some inactive ingredients like cedar leaf oil, nutmeg oil, petroleum oil, thymol and turpentine oil, which are indicated as over-the-counter ointments to suppress cough in patients above 2 years. Recently, some of these components have shown efficacy against dermatophytes in vitro.[25] Thus, they have been popularized as home remedies for fungal nail infections although there is lack of definite evidence.

In vitro studies have shown antifungal activity against *C. albicans*, most notably for camphor, menthol, thymol and eucalyptus oil.[8] Fungal cell membrane damage and inhibition of germ tube synthesis are the probable mechanisms.

There is a single pilot study involving 85 patients who applied TCS once daily to the affected nails. Approximately 38% showed complete remission, maximum after 9 months, with once daily application. No adverse effects have been reported.[8] Thus, further studies are needed to recommend its clinical usage.

Natural Coniferous Resin Lacquer[8]

Natural coniferous resin (NCR), obtained from the Norway spruce tree, has been used since centuries in the Scandinavian countries to treat superficial wounds and infections. In vitro studies have demonstrated broad-spectrum activity of NCR against both gram-positive bacteria and fungi. Plate diffusion studies have confirmed its effectiveness against *Trichophyton*, but not against *Fusarium* or *Candida*.

There are two published clinical trials evaluating NCR in the treatment of onychomycosis. The first trial involving 15 participants demonstrated mycological cure in 65% subjects, while none showed clinical cure; at the end of 9 months. The second study was a comparative trial, 13% showed mycological cure in the NCR group compared to 8% and 56% in the amorolfine and terbinafine groups. Approximately 30% patients in the NCR group showed partial clinical improvement. None of the patients in the NCR group had any adverse effect, and cost of therapy was minimum for this group. Thus, NCR lacquer may be considered a safe and cost-effective over-the-counter adjunctive therapy for onychomycosis.

Ageratina pichinchensis Extract

Ageratina pichinchensis extract, obtained from plants of the Asteraceae family, has been historically used in Mexico for the treatment of superficial fungal infections. Multiple clinical trials have demonstrated the efficacy of this substance in tinea pedis both clinically and mycologically. Thus, the role of this agent was investigated in onychomycosis.

In vitro data shows maximum efficacy against the dermatophytes *T. rubrum* and *T. mentagrophytes*, mainly fungotoxic action.

A single doubly blind controlled trial has shown comparable efficacy in mild-to-moderate toenail onychomycosis in comparison to ciclopirox nail lacquer. *A. pichinchensis* extract was applied once twice weekly for the first 2 months, followed by weekly application for the next 16 weeks. No severe adverse effect has been reported except minimal periungual pain in 2.7% patients.[26]

Ozonized Sunflower Oil

Ozonized sunflower oil is prepared by passing ozone (O_3) through sunflower oil to form a petroleum jelly-like material. It has antibacterial, anti-inflammatory, antifungal and wound-healing properties.

In vitro studies have demonstrated growth inhibition of *C. albicans*, *C. parapsilosis* and *C. tropicalis*; however being inferior to amphotericin B and the azoles.[8]

A single-blind, controlled phase III trial has shown considerable efficacy and reduced relapse rate post-therapy, compared to ketoconazole 2% cream. No notable adverse effect has been reported.[8]

CONCLUSION

Onychomycosis is a chronic persistent condition, which requires treatment for a long duration, topical modality being an important component. Although there are several approved topical antifungals, longer treatment duration, slow clinical improvement, high cost of therapy along with systemic adverse effects often act as deterrents. Lately, there is a renewed interest in several natural remedies, to bridge this gap. However, the later agents can be used as adjuvants at best. Proper patient counseling regarding weekly nail trimming and nail filing is of paramount importance to obtain best results.

REFERENCES

1. Gupta AK, Gupta G, Jain HC, Lynde CW, Foley KA, Daigle D, et al. The prevalence of unsuspected onychomycosis and its causative organisms in a multicentre Canadian sample of 30,000 patients visiting physicians' offices. *J Eur Acad Dermatol Venereol.* 2016;30:1567-72.
2. Scher RK, Rich P, Pariser D, Elewski B. The epidemiology, etiology, and pathophysiology of onychomycosis. *Semin Cutan Med Surg.* 2013;32(2 Suppl 1):S2-4.
3. Lipner SR, Scher RK. Onychomycosis: topical therapy and devices. In: Rubin AI, Jellinek NJ, Daniel CR, Scher RK (Eds). Scher and Daniel's Nails: Diagnosis, Surgery, Therapy. Philadelphia: Springer Nature, 2018. pp. 173-83.
4. Lecha M, Effendy I, Feuilhade de Chauvin M, Di Chiacchio N, Baran R. Treatment options—development of consensus guidelines. *J Eur Acad Dermatol Venereol.* 2005;19 Suppl 1:25-33.
5. Angelo T, Borgheti-Cardoso LN, Gelfuso GM, Taveira SF, Gratieri T. Chemical and physical strategies in onychomycosis topical treatment: a review. *Med Mycol.* 2017;55(5):461-75.
6. Burkhart CN, Burkhart CG, Gupta AK. Dermatophytoma: recalcitrance to treatment because of existence of fungal biofilm. *J Am Acad Dermatol.* 2002;47:629-31.
7. Akhtar N, Sharma H, Pathak K. Onychomycosis: potential of nail lacquers in transungual delivery of antifungals. *Scientifica (Cairo).* 2016;2016:1387936.
8. Halteh P, Scher RK, Lipner SR. Over-the-counter and natural remedies for onychomycosis: do they really work? *Cutis.* 2016;98(5):E16-25.
9. Bohn M, Kraemer KT. Dermatopharmacology of ciclopirox nail lacquer topical solution 8% in the treatment of onychomycosis. *J Am Acad Dermatol.* 2000;43(4 Suppl):S57-69.
10. Subissi A, Monti D, Togni G, Mailland F. Ciclopirox: recent nonclinical and clinical data relevant to its use as a topical antimycotic agent. *Drugs.* 2010;70(16):2133-52.
11. Gupta AK, Fleckman P, Baran R. Ciclopirox nail lacquer topical solution 8% in the treatment of toenail onychomycosis. *J Am Acad Dermatol.* 2000;43(4 suppl):S70-80.
12. Polak A. Preclinical data and mode of action of amorolfine. *Dermatology.* 1992;184 Suppl 1:3-7.
13. Haria M, Bryson HM. Amorolfine: a review of its pharmacological properties and therapeutic potential in the treatment of onychomycosis and other superficial fungal infections. *Drugs.* 1995;49:103-20.
14. Franz TJ. Absorption of amorolfine through human nail. *Dermatology.* 1992;184(Suppl 1):18-20.
15. Sigurgeirsson B, Olafsson JH, Steinsson JT, Kerrouche N, Sidou F. Efficacy of amorolfine nail lacquer for the prophylaxis of onychomycosis over 3 years. *J Eur Acad Dermatol Venereol.* 2010;24:910-5.
16. Elewski BE, Rich P, Pollak R, et al. Efinaconazole 10% solution in the treatment of toenail onychomycosis: two phase III multicenter, randomized, double-blind studies. *J Am Acad Dermatol.* 2013;68(4):600-8.
17. Sugiura K, Sugimoto N, Hosaka S, et al. The low keratin affinity of efinaconazole contributes to its nail penetration and fungicidal activity in topical onychomycosis treatment. *Antimicrob Agents Chemother.* 2014;58(7):3837-42.
18. Gupta AK, Cernea M. How effective is efinaconazole in the management of onychomycosis? *Expert Opin Pharmacother.* 2016;17(4):611-8.
19. Iwata A, Watanabe Y, Kumagai N, et al. In vitro and in vivo assessment of dermatophyte acquired resistance to efinaconazole, a novel triazole antifungal. *Antimicrob Agents Chemother.* 2014;58(8):4920-2.
20. Sharma N, Sharma D. An upcoming drug for onychomycosis: tavaborole. *J Pharmacol Pharmacother.* 2015;6(4):236-9.

21. Elewski BE, Aly R, Baldwin SL, et al. Efficacy and safety of tavaborole topical solution, 5%, a novel boron-based antifungal agent, for the treatment of toenail onychomycosis: results from 2 randomized phase-III studies. *J Am Acad Dermatol*. 2015;73:62-9.
22. Concha JM, Moore LS, Holloway WJ. 1998 William J. Stickel Bronze Award. Antifungal activity of Melaleuca alternifolia (tea-tree) oil against various pathogenic organisms. *J Am Podiatr Med Assoc*. 1998;88:489-92.
23. Buck DS, Nidorf DM, Addino JG. Comparison of two topical preparations for the treatment of onychomycosis: Melaleuca alternifolia (tea tree) oil and clotrimazole. *J Fam Pract*. 1994;38:601-5.
24. Syed TA, Qureshi ZA, Ali SM, Ahmad S, Ahmad SA. Treatment of toenail onychomycosis with 2% butenafine and 5% Melaleuca alternifolia (tea tree) oil in cream. *Trop Med Int Health*. 1999;4:284-7.
25. Pinto E, Pina-Vaz C, Salgueiro L, et al. Antifungal activity of the essential oil of Thymus pulegioides on Candida, Aspergillus and dermatophyte species. *J Med Microbiol*. 2006;55:1367-73.
26. Romero-Cerecero O, Zamilpa A, Jimenez-Ferrer JE, et al. Double-blind clinical trial for evaluating the effectiveness and tolerability of Ageratina pichinchensis extract on patients with mild to moderate onychomycosis. A comparative study with ciclopirox. *Planta Med*. 2008;74:1430-5.

World Clin Dermatol. 2019;5(1):57-67.

Topical Polyenes

*Mala Bhalla MD, Monika MD

Department of Dermatology, Venereology and Leprosy,
Government Medical College and Hospital, Chandigarh, Punjab, India

ABSTRACT

Topical polyenes represent a group of antifungals which have been used successfully in the management of various superficial cutaneous and mucocutaneous infections. Nystatin and amphotericin B are readily available topical polyenes. Several newer formulations of topical polyenes have been recently introduced with improved efficacy and safety profile. They seem to be a potential alternative in recalcitrant superficial infections of skin in the current scenario of antifungal resistance though their indiscriminate use should be discouraged. This article focuses on topical polyenes and their clinical uses in the field of dermatology.

INTRODUCTION

Superficial fungal infections are an important cause of morbidity. The most common amongst superficial fungal infections is dermatophytoses resulting from fungi that affect the keratinized tissues of the skin, hair and nails. Skin commensal yeasts, such as *Malassezia furfur*, *Candida* species, *Aspergillus* are other important fungi causing superficial infection of skin.[1]

Treatment of dermatomycoses can be in the form of systemic or topical antifungals. Topical antifungals play an important role as adjuvants in treatment of dermatophytosis, however, they may also be used alone in localized superficial infections. The efficacy of topical agents in superficial fungal infections depends on penetrability of drug into the affected tissue and potency of drug against various fungi.[2]

---

*Corresponding author
Email: malabhalla@yahoo.co. in

On the basis of their mechanism of action, topical antifungal agents can be divided into various groups: (1) azoles (2) allylamines (3) polyenes (4) miscellaneous like morpholines, ciclopirox olamine, selenium sulfide, zinc pyrithione, oxaboroles and tolnaftate, etc. Polyene, the oldest antifungals, are heterocyclic antibiotics derived from *Streptomyces* species.[3] Various polyene antifungals include amphotericin B, nystatin, candicidin, natamycin, perimycin, ascosin, hamycin, endomycin, candihexin, dermostatin, eurocidin, fungichromatin, flavomycoin, rimocidin and etruscomycin. They have been extensively used in the treatment of topical and systemic fungal infections caused by *Candida, Fusarium, Mucor, Aspergillus, Rhizopus, Scedosporium, Trichosporon, Cryptococcus* as well as in parasitic infections such as leishmaniasis and amebiasis. However, as the systemic use of polyenes is associated with many severe adverse effects such as nephrotoxicity, hepatotoxicity and hematologic side effects, their systemic use is restricted to life-threatening invasive infections and certain agents are primarily used as topical agents only. Despite a large number of polyene molecules available, the topically available agents are only a few which include nystatin, amphotericin B, candicidin, natamycin and hamycin. These drugs are available as various formulations such as creams, ointment, gel, powder, pessaries, etc., with recent introduction of few newer advanced formulations.

CHEMICAL STRUCTURE OF POLYENES

These are cyclic amphipathic molecules characterized by three basic structural components—a polyene and a polyol chain that together constitute a macrolide ring, and a mycosamine substituent (Figures 1 to 4).[4] Nystatin and amphotericin B have a great structural similarity with the differentiating points being:

- Number of conjugated double bonds, nystatin is a tetraene (four double bonds) while amphotericin B is heptaene (seven double bonds);
- Different distributions of the hydroxyl groups in the polyol chain
- Interruption of the conjugated double bonds in the case of nystatin.[4]

Polyenes enter the fungal membranes containing ergosterol, forming a pore that leads to leakage of cellular compounds, elimination of ion and electrical gradients, and ultimately cell death.[5] Topical polyene antibiotics also have surface-active properties allowing them to spread at surfaces, hence, making them ideal drugs for topical application. These are available in different concentrations and compounded into conventional, as well as newer vehicles, thereby, increasing efficacy and decreasing local irritancy (Table 1). They show rapid degradation under the influence of light but the heptaene amphotericin B is more photostable than the tetraenes nystatin and natamycin.

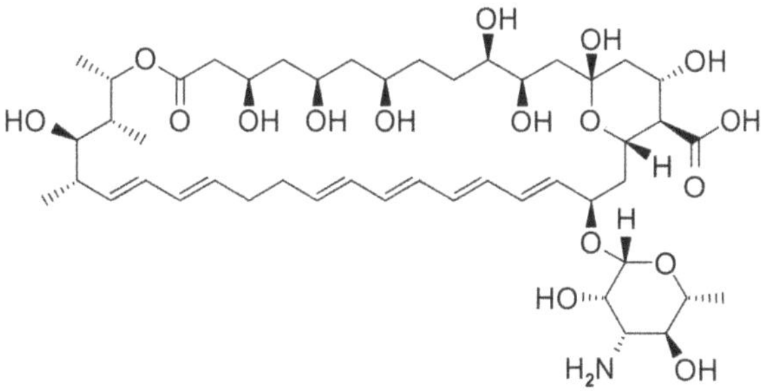

Figure 1: Structure of nystatin.

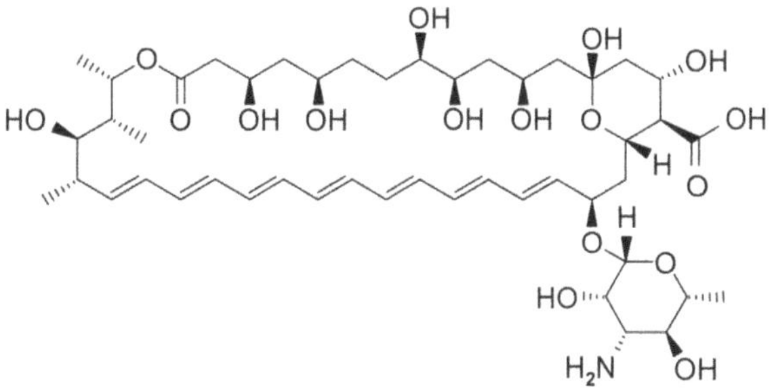

Figure 2: Structure of amphotericin B.

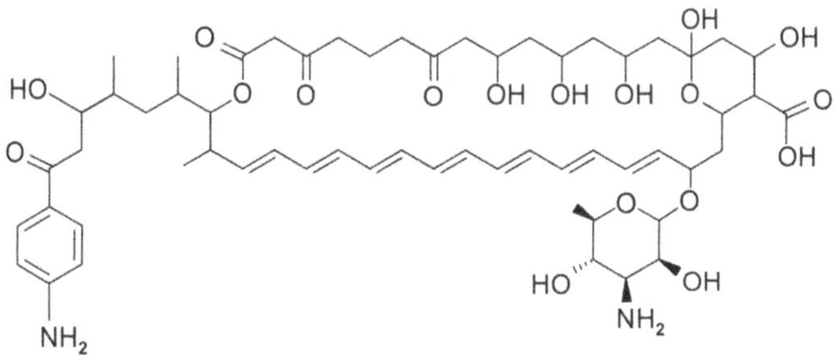

Figure 3: Structure of candicidin.

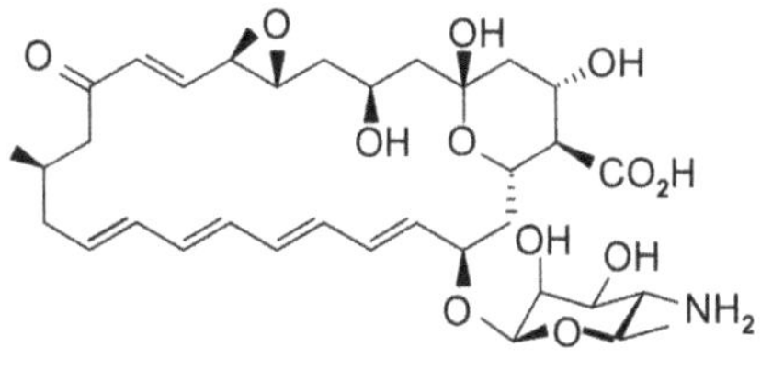

Figure 4: Structure of natamycin.

Table 1: List of Topical Polyenes and their Formulations		
Drug	**Available concentration and formulations**	**Frequency of application**
Nystatin	• Cream/ointment (100,000 U/g) • Lozenge (200,000 U) • Powder (100,000 U/g) • Vaginal cream (25,000 U/g) • Vaginal tablet (100,000 U)	Twice daily for cutaneous fungal infections and three to four times for mucocutaneous infections for 2–3 weeks
Amphotericin B	• Liposomal 0.1% gel • 3% cream • 0.15% eye drops	Twice daily for 2–4 weeks
Natamycin	• 2% vaginal cream • 5% ophthalmic solution	-
Candicidin	• Vaginal ointment	-
Hamycin	• Vaginal pessary/cream • Oral suspension—200,000 IU/mL	-

HISTORY OF POLYENES

Brown and Hazen, in 1948, first observed the antifungal effect of a substance produced by soil actinomycete which led to the discovery of first polyene named as nystatin.[3] Since this date, there have been many published reports of polyene antifungals; it is difficult to determine the exact total number, with a rough estimation being around hundred. Polyenes are almost exclusively produced by Streptomycetaceae group of bacteria, mainly by *Streptomyces* species and *Streptoverticillium* species.[6] Two years later, in 1950, Nystatin was isolated from *Streptomyces albidus* and *Streptomyces noursei*. Initially, it was named as fungicidin, which was later renamed to nystatin based on the New York State, where both researchers worked.[7] In 1956, a new compound, amphotericin B was isolated by Gold and colleagues, from a filamentous bacterium, *Streptomyces nodosus*. Since then, polyenes have remained a gold standard for the treatment of cutaneous and systemic fungal infections.[8]

MECHANISM OF ACTION

Polyenes act by forming a complex with ergosterol in the plasma membrane of fungus, causing membrane disruption leading to increased permeability and leakage of cytoplasmic contents, and ultimately cell death.[9,10] Further experiments are still being performed on the influence of polyenes on natural membrane properties and pores formation.[11,12] The radius of pore-forming complex is influenced by the structure of polyenes, e.g. amphotericin B forms larger transmembrane pores which allows the leakage of intracellular ions as well as larger molecules whereas nystatin forms smaller transmembrane pores, through which only intracellular ions and smaller molecules, such as glucose, can pass.[13]

Polyenes have higher affinity for fungal cell membrane ergosterol than mammalian cell membranes which are characterized by cholesterol as the major sterol. This may be attributed to the difference in the chemical structure of ergosterol and cholesterol as the former has more number of double bonds which allow the stronger van der Waals interactions with polyenes. On the contrary, due to the absence of double bonds in cholesterol, its conformational stability decreases thus making its interaction with polyenes less amenable. Polyenes have also been found to trigger free radical induced oxidative damage to cells and inhibit the cell membrane transport of amino acids and glucose.[14]

There is some evidence that polyenes do not exert their fungicidal effect primarily by insertion of pore forming complexes in fungal cell membranes, rather, the pores are formed secondarily following their interaction with ergosterol which leads to a disturbance in membrane signaling pathways and process of endocytosis.

SPECTRUM OF ACTIVITY

Unlike systemic polyenes which possess broad-spectrum of activity against many pathogenic and opportunistic fungi, the topical polyenes exhibit a limited in vitro activity against fewer fungal pathogens. Topical nystatin shows both in vitro fungistatic and fungicidal activity against *Candida* species such as *Candida albicans, Candida tropicalis, Candida parapsilosis* and *Candida krusei*. Nystatin has no inhibitory effects on dermatophytic strains, hence, not indicated for dermatophytosis.

Topical amphotericin B shows potent in vitro antifungal activity against dermatophytic strains of *Trichophyton, Microsporum* and *Epidermophyton* genera, *Candida* species, *Trichosporon, Saccharomyces* species, *Leishmania donovani, Trypanosoma* species and *Sporothrix schenkii*.[3]

Nystatin

Pharmacology

Nystatin is the oldest polyene antifungal agent, isolated from a bacterium, *S. nodosus*.[3] Because of its poor oral bioavailability and toxicity following parenteral administration, nystatin is mainly limited to topical use. The percutaneous absorption of nystatin is almost negligible.

Spectrum of Activity

Nystatin shows in vitro antifungal activity against most *Candida* species such as *C. albicans*, *C. tropicalis*, *C. parapsilosis* and *C. krusei*.[15] Nystatin does not possess much activity against dermatophytes, bacteria, protozoa, or viruses.

Clinical Use

Nystatin is commercially available as a cream or ointment (100,000 U/g), lozenge (200,000 U) and powder (100,000 U/g). Twice daily application is required for cutaneous infections and four to five times daily use is recommended in oral candidiasis as slowly dissolving pastille formulations have been used effectively.[16] It is also available as a vaginal cream (25,000 U/g) and vaginal tablet (100,000 U) for the treatment of vaginal candidiasis, in the recommended dose of once daily at bed time for 2 weeks. Recently, the nanocapsular hydrogel loaded with nystatin has been introduced as a promising dosage form for the treatment of cutaneous candidiasis.[17] It has been formulated to avoid undesirable side effects of systemic absorption and toxicity.[18] It is clinically ineffective in the treatment of dermatophytosis.

Pregnancy category—Category B.

Amphotericin B

Pharmacology

Amphotericin B is a polyene antifungal agent with seven conjugated double bonds in its macrolactone ring, produced by *S. nodosus*. There are two forms—amphotericin A and B out of which amphotericin A is not used clinically. Initially, amphotericin B was compounded into cream, gel, lotion and ointment forms for its use in cutaneous mycoses but due to high lipophilicity and poor aqueous solubility, these conventional formulations had limited efficacy, even at higher doses and were rather associated with several adverse reactions such as pruritus, redness, peeling, dryness, irritation and severe blistering of the skin.[19] To overcome these drawbacks, newer vehicles for amphotericin B were explored and evaluated, of which lipid-based carrier systems were a major therapeutic success. These lipid carriers increase the lipophilicity, hence, allows better penetration of the drug into the target tissues and reduces the risk of local adverse effects.[20] Liposomal gel, solid lipid nanoparticles (SLNs) and microemulsion gel are few of the newer formulations of amphotericin B being used for the management of superficial infections of skin. Following topical application of liposomal-based gel, a major fraction (about 90%) is released within 2 hours, thus, providing a rapid therapeutic effect.

Spectrum of Activity

Topical amphotericin B shows in vitro antifungal activity against most dermatophytes *Candida* species, *Trichosporon, Saccharomyces* species, *Trypanosoma* species and *S. schenkii*.[3] It has been shown to inhibit the morphogenetic transformation of *C. albicans* at concentration close to minimum inhibitory concentration (MIC). It also possesses leishmanicidal activity with low incidence of clinical resistance.

Clinical Use

Liposomal amphotericin B is commercially available as 0.1% liposomal gel and 0.1% nanoemulsion gel. It has been used effectively for the treatment of cutaneous fungal infections such as cutaneous candidiasis, dermatophytosis and cutaneous leishmaniasis.[21] Liposomal amphotericin B in adjunct with thermotherapy has been proved to be efficacious in the management of fixed cutaneous sporotrichosis, in the dose of twice daily application resulting in complete healing in 8 weeks.[22]

Though it possesses potent antifungal activity against dermatophytes, amphotericin B is not generally considered as topical agent of choice for dermatophytosis. Its use is usually reserved for the recalcitrant dermatophytic infections responding poorly to commonly used topical agents such as azoles and allylamines. Of note, the irrational use of amphotericin B should be avoided in dermatophytosis as this would otherwise be associated with a potential risk of clinical resistance.

Mycotic corneal ulcer and keratitis can be cured with topical drops, as well as by direct subconjunctival injection. Amphotericin B has been used successfully to treat epithelial keratitis due to *Rhodotomla* species and fungal endopthalmitis. Recently, a microneedle-based delivery of amphotericin B has been investigated for cutaneous leishmaniasis in murine models.[23]

Pregnancy category—Category B.

Natamycin

Pharmacology

Natamycin (earlier called as Pimaricin) is a tetraene polyene antifungal derived from *Streptomyces natalensis*. It was discovered in 1955 and approved for medical use in the United States in 1978.[24] Natamycin has a poor aqueous solubility.

Spectrum of Activity

It has been shown to inhibit variety of yeasts including *Candida* and filamentous fungi including *Aspergillus* species, *Fusarium* species, *Cephalosporium, Penicillium,*

Trichomonas and *Leishmania* species. Its MIC is very low (<10 ppm) for most of the filamentous fungi.

Clinical Use

It is available as 2% cream for the treatment of candidial vaginitis, trichomonal vaginitis, nonspecific vaginitis, cutaneous infections due to *Candida* and *Aspergillus* species.[25] It is widely used as 5% ophthalmic suspension for the treatment of mycotic keratitis.[26] Natamycin lozenges are also used for the treatment of oral thrush. It is also used in the food industry as a preservative.

Pregnancy category—Category C.

Candicidin

Pharmacology

Candicidin is a heptaene polyene macrolide complex, obtained from *Streptomyces griseus*. The antibiotic complex is composed of candicidins A, B, C and D, of which D is the major component. The name "Candicidin" was given due to its high activity on *C. albicans*. Its antifungal activity is markedly influenced by pH unlike other polyenes which are least affected by alteration in pH.[27]

Spectrum of Activity

It has demonstrated to be active against most *Candida* species, *Streptomyces* and filamentous fungi like *Aspergillus*.

Clinical Use

Candicidin has been used extensively for successful treatment of candidal vulvovaginitis and cutaneous forms of candidiasis including intertriginous and paronychial moniliasis.[28]

Hamycin

Pharmacology

Hamycin is heptaene polyene derived from *Streptomyces pimprina*. It was first isolated in India by Thirumalachar et al. in 1961. The chemical structure of hamycin is similar to amphotericin B except the presence of an additional aromatic ring attached to the molecule.

Spectrum of Activity

It has been shown to be effective against *Candida*, *Malassezia ovale* and *Trichomonas*.

Clinical Use

Hamycin is available as oral suspension (200,000 IU/mL) and vaginal pessary. It is produced by only one company, Hindustan Antibiotics Ltd. It has been used for the treatment of trichomonas vaginalis, vaginal moniliasis and oral candidiasis.

ADVERSE EFFECTS OF TOPICAL POLYENES

Topical polyenes are generally well-tolerated by patients. Less commonly, minor and transient adverse effects have been reported like burning, pruritus, eczema and pain on application. Allergic contact dermatitis to parent compound or vehicle such as propylene glycol or sodium sulfite can also occur rarely. Very rarely transaminitis, pyuria and hematuria have been reported with the use of amphotericin gel.[21]

CONTRAINDICATIONS

Hypersensitivity to parent compound or any of constituents of formulation.

TOPICAL POLYENES IN SPECIAL SITUATIONS

Nystatin and amphotericin B both are category B in pregnancy. However, with the use of topical nystatin, recent Hungarian data raised the possibility of slightly increased chances of hypospadias in exposed fetuses.[29] All may be safely used in lactation, as there is minimal secretion in breast milk.

EMERGING TRENDS IN TOPICAL POLYENES

- *Use of newer formulations/vehicles*:
  - Lipid-based amphotericin B gel: Better penetration and therapeutic efficacy, lesser chances of local irritancy
  - Amphotericin B-Cyclodextrins methyl cellulose gel: Cyclodextrins have inhibitory effect on biofilm formation, thus, enhancing the topical penetration of amphotericin B by acting as solubilizers and stabilizer agents. Among cyclodextrins, gamma-cyclodextrins have the highest aqueous solubility and biggest cavity when compared to other parental cyclodextrins[30,31]

- o Amphotericin B microemulsion: Microemulsion formulation helps in increasing drug penetration and lowering local irritancy.[32]
- *Microneedle–based delivery of amphotericin*: This enhances the drug penetration and has been shown to have good results in the treatment of small nodules caused by *Leishmania mexicana*. It is not much effective for the disseminated infection. However, further studies are needed to establish it as an optimized method of drug delivery.[23]

CONCLUSION

Topical polyenes have a critical role to play in the management of cutaneous mycoses. Newer topical antifungals and specialized formulations do hold a lot of promise in the future in the management of superficial fungal as well as other cutaneous infections.[33]

REFERENCES

1. Borgers M, Degreef H, Cauwenbergh G. Fungal infections of the skin: infection process and antimycotic therapy. *Curr Drug Targets*. 2005;6(8):849-62.
2. Erbagci Z. Topical therapy for dermatophytoses: should corticosteroids be included? *Am J Clin Dermatol*. 2004;5(6):375-84.
3. Hammond SM. Biological activity of polyene antibiotics. *Prog Med Chem*. 1977;14:105-79.
4. Kristanc L, Božič B, Jokhadar ŠZ, Dolenc MS, Gomišček G. The pore-forming action of polyenes: From model membranes to living organisms. *Biochim Biophys Acta Biomembr*. 2019;1861(2):418-30.
5. Hac-Wydro K, Dynarowicz-Latka P. Interaction between nystatin and natural membrane lipids in Langmuir monolayers—the role of a phospholipid in the mechanism of polyenes mode of action. *Biophys Chem*. 2006;123(2-3):154-61.
6. Waksman SA. The actinomycetes and their antibiotics. *Adv Appl Microbiol*. 1963;5:235-315.
7. Brown R, Hazen EL. Activation of antifungal extracts of actinomycetes by ultrafiltration through gradocol membranes. *Proc Soc Exp Biol Med*. 1949;71(3):454-7.
8. Donovick R, Gold W, Pagano JF, Stout HA. Amphotericins A and B, antifungal antibiotics produced by a streptomycete. I. In vitro studies. *Antibiot Annu*. 1955-1656;3:579-86.
9. Cheah HL, Lim V, Sandai D. Inhibitors of the glyoxylate cycle enzyme ICL1 in *Candida albicans* for potential use as antifungal agents. *PloS One*. 2014;9(4):e95951.
10. Gallis HA, Drew RH, Pickard WW. Amphotericin B: 30 years of clinical experience. *Rev Infect Dis*. 1990;12(2):308-29.
11. Carrillo-Muñoz AJ, Quindós G, Tur C, Ruesga MT, Miranda Y, del Valle O, et al. In-vitro antifungal activity of liposomal nystatin in comparison with nystatin, amphotericin B cholesteryl sulphate, liposomal amphotericin B, amphotericin B lipid complex, amphotericin B desoxycholate, fluconazole and itraconazole. *J Antimicrob Chemother*. 1999;44(3):397-401.
12. Ostrosky-Zeichner L, Bazemore S, Paetznick VL, Rodriguez JR, Chen E, Wallace T, et al. Differential antifungal activity of isomeric forms of nystatin. *Antimicrob Agents Chemother*. 2001;45(10):2781-6.
13. Cohen BE. Amphotericin B membrane action: role for two types of ion channels in eliciting cell survival and lethal effects. *J Membr Biol*. 2010;238(1-3):1-20.
14. Efimova SS, Schagina LV, Ostroumova OS. Investigation of channel-forming activity of polyene macrolide antibiotics in planar lipid bilayers in the presence of dipole modifiers. *Acta Naturae*. 2014;6(4):67-79.

15. Kuriyama T, Williams DW, Bagg J, Coulter WA, Ready D, Lewis MA. In vitro susceptibility of oral Candida to seven antifungal agents. *Oral Microbiol Immunol*. 2005;20(6):349-53.
16. Dias MF, Bernardes-Filho F, Quaresma-Santos MV, Amorim AG, Schechtman RC, Azulay DR. Treatment of superficial mycoses: review. Part II. *An Bras Dermatol*. 2013;88(6):937-44.
17. AbouSamra MM, Basha M, Awad GE, Mansy SS. A promising nystatin nanocapsular hydrogel as an antifungal polymeric carrier for the treatment of topical candidiasis. *J Drug Deliv Sci Technol*. 2019;49:365-74.
18. Elmoslemany RM, Abdallah OY, El-Khordagui LK, Khalafallah NM. Propylene glycol liposomes as a topical delivery system for miconazole nitrate: comparison with conventional liposomes. *AAPS Pharm Sci Tech*. 2012;13(2):723-31.
19. Devi M, Kumar MS, Mahadevan N. Amphotericin-B loaded vesicular systems for the treatment of topical fungal infection. *Int J Recent Adv Pharm*. 2011;4:37-46.
20. Müller RH, Radtke M, Wissing SA. Solid lipid nanoparticles (SLN) and nanostructured lipid carriers (NLC) in cosmetic and dermatological preparations. *Adv Drug Deliv Rev*. 2002;54(Suppl 1):S131-55.
21. Sheikh S, Ali SM, Ahmad MU, Ahmad A, Mushtaq M, Paithankar M, et al. Nanosomal amphotericin B is an efficacious alternative to ambisome for fungal therapy. *Int J Pharm*. 2010;397(1-2):103-8.
22. Mahajan VK, Mehta KS, Chauhan PS, Gupta M, Sharma R, Rawat R. Fixed cutaneous sporotrichosis treated with topical amphotericin B in an immune suppressed patient. *Med Mycol Case Rep*. 2015;7:23-5.
23. Nguyen AK, Yang KH, Bryant K, Li J, Joice AC, Werbovetz KA, et al. Microneedle-based delivery of amphotericin B for treatment of cutaneous leishmaniasis. *Biomed Microdevices*. 2019;21(1):8.
24. Thrum H. W. P. RAAB, Natamycin (Pimaricin). Its Properties and Possibilities in Medicine. 134 S., 23 Abb., 37 Tab. Stuttgart-New York 1972: Georg Thieme Publishers - Intercontinental Medical Book Corp. DM 19,80. *Z Allg Mikrobiol*. 1974;14(2):172.
25. Buch A, Skytte Christensen E. Treatment of vaginal candidosis with natamycin and effect of treating the partner at the same time. *Acta Obstet Gynecol Scand*. 1982;61(5):393-6.
26. Sharma N, Singhal D, Maharana PK, Sinha R, Agarwal T, Upadhyay AD, et al. Comparison of oral voriconazole versus oral ketoconazole as an adjunct to topical natamycin in severe fungal keratitis: a randomized controlled trial. *Cornea*. 2017;36(12):1521-7.
27. Padhye AA, Thirumalachar MJ. Hamycin in the treatment of *Cryptococcus neoformans* in mice. *Hindustan Antibiot Bull*. 1963;6:41-3.
28. Morese KN. Candicidin tablets and ointment in treatment of candidal vaginitis. *N Y State J Med*. 1975;75(9):1443-5.
29. Pilmis B, Jullien V, Sobel J, Lecuit M, Lortholary O, Charlier C. Antifungal drugs during pregnancy: an updated review. *J Antimicrob Chemother*. 2015;70(1):14-22.
30. López-Castillo C, Rodríguez-Fernández C, Córdoba M, Torrado JJ. Permeability characteristics of a new antifungal topical amphotericin B formulation with γ-cyclodextrins. *Molecules*. 2018;23(12):3349.
31. Ruiz HK, Serrano DR, Dea-Ayuela MA, Bilbao-Ramos PE, Bolás-Fernández F, Torrado JJ, et al. New amphotericin B-gamma-cyclodextrin formulation for topical use with synergistic activity against diverse fungal species and *Leishmania* spp. *Int J Pharm*. 2014;473(1-2):148-57.
32. Butani D, Yewale C, Misra A. Amphotericin B topical microemulsion: Formulation, characterization and evaluation. *Colloids Surf B Biointerfaces*. 2014;116:351-8.
33. Poojary SA. Topical antifungals: a review and their role in current management of dermatophytoses. *Clin Dermatol Rev*. 2017;1(3):24-9.

World Clin Dermatol. 2019;5(1):68-81.

Allylamine and Benzylamine Topical Antifungals

[1,*]Nisha V Parmar MD, [2]Rashmi Sarkar MD MNAMS

[1]Department of Dermatology, Rashid Hospital,
Dubai Health Authority, Dubai, United Arab Emirates
[2]Department of Dermatology, STD and Leprosy, Maulana Azad Medical
College and Lok Nayak Hospital, New Delhi, India

ABSTRACT

The allylamines and benzylamine antifungals are a relatively new class of topical antifungal agents. They act by inhibiting squalene epoxidase enzyme, the rate-limiting enzyme in fungal cell membrane synthesis. These agents, thus, have enhanced antifungal activity due to the fact that they are fungicidal and also possess anti-inflammatory properties. This article discusses in detail the role of topical allylamine and benzylamine antifungal agents in the management of superficial fungal infections.

INTRODUCTION

The allylamine and benzylamine group of antifungal agents were discovered in the 1970s, 1980s and 1990s. The topical allylamines include naftifine and terbinafine, and butenafine is the sole topical benzylamine. Squalene epoxidase inhibition, a mechanism independent from the inhibition of the cytochrome p450-related enzyme lanosterol-14α-demethylase through which the azole antifungals act, confers a superior efficacy to this class of drugs. Currently, topical allylamines and benzylamine are the first choice antifungal agents for the treatment of dermatophytic infections.

*Corresponding author
Email: parmarnish@gmail.com

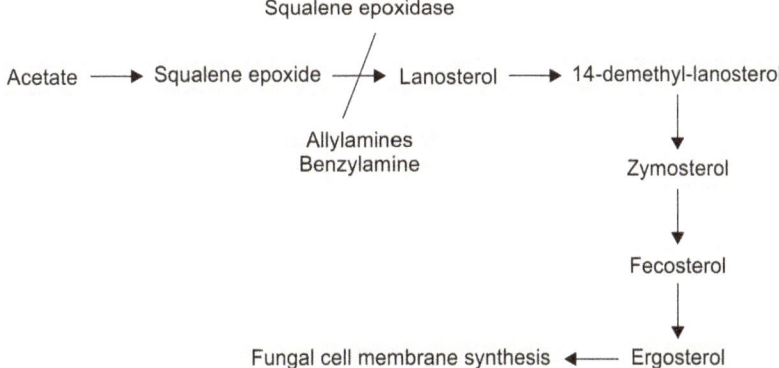

Figure 1: Mechanism of action of allylamines and benzylamine.

ALLYLAMINES

The discovery of allylamine antifungals was a milestone in antifungal treatment as they possess fungicidal properties in addition to their fungistatic activity. Allylamines block ergosterol synthesis by inhibiting the rate-limiting enzyme, squalene epoxidase (Figure 1). Ergosterol is the chief component of fungal cell membrane. Blockage of squalene epoxidase leads to accumulation of squalene and subsequent intracellular changes that lead to the death of the fungi. Allylamines have a broad-spectrum of antifungal activity aimed at dermatophytes, molds and yeasts.

NAFTIFINE

Naftifine is the first member of the allylamine group of antifungals to be discovered. In 1974, research aimed at finding an active antifungal compound targeting the central nervous system at the Sandoz Research Institute in Vienna, Austria led to the serendipitous discovery of naftifine.[1]

Chemistry

Naftifine is a synthetic allylamine which exists as a crystalline lightly yellow powder. Its chemical formula is $C21H21N$ (Figure 2).

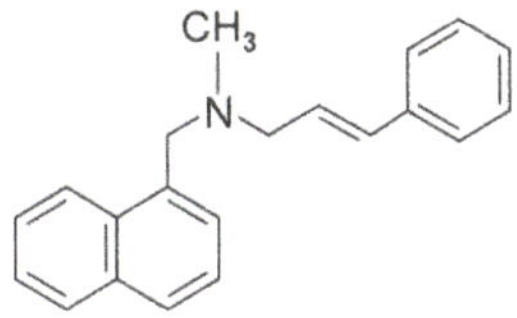

Figure 2: Chemical structure of naftifine.

Mechanism of Action

Antifungal Activity

Naftifine inhibits squalene epoxidase, the rate-limiting enzyme in ergosterol synthesis. Inhibition of squalene epoxidase leads to intracellular accumulation of squalene which results in multiple intracellular degenerative processes such as lipid accumulation in the cytoplasm as well as the endoplasmic reticulum. Lack of squalene downstream leads to cessation of ergosterol and subsequent fungal cell membrane synthesis demonstrating the fungistatic action. A combination of lack of ergosterol and accumulation of intracellular lipid droplets ultimately causes destruction of the fungus, hence, accounting for the fungicidal action of naftifine.

Naftifine was found to be chiefly fungicidal against dermatophytes and molds. Concerning yeasts, naftifine is chiefly fungistatic except for *Candida parapsilosis* against which it is fungicidal.[1]

Naftifine was found to demonstrate the maximum antifungal activity at a neutral pH.[1]

Antibacterial Activity

Naftifine has significant antibacterial property targeted against both gram-positive as well as gram-negative bacteria including—*Staphylococcus aureus*, *Streptococcus pyogenes*, *Pseudomonas aeruginosa*, *Escherichia coli* and a few *Corynebacterium* species.

Anti-inflammatory Activity

Few studies have demonstrated the anti-inflammatory role of naftifine 1% cream in the treatment of dermatophytoses. In a double blinded randomized controlled trial comparing 1% naftifine cream versus 1% clotrimazole plus 1% hydrocortisone cream in 115 patients with proven fungal infection of the skin, both treatments were found to be equally effective. The study concluded that naftifine has an anti-inflammatory effect equal to clotrimazole-hydrocortisone combination.[2]

Pharmacodynamics and Pharmacokinetics

Naftifine takes the transdermal route of penetration to reach its site of action, the stratum corneum. Its penetration into the various layers of the skin was studied through in vitro testing of 14C-labeled naftifine. This experiment found the following levels of naftifine in the respective layers—1,300 µg/mL in the stratum corneum, 38 µg/mL in the other layers of the epidermis, 13.5 µg/mL in the dermis and 0.5 µg/mL in the subcutis.[3] A similar experiment was performed in the layers of the nail and naftifine was found in all layers of the nail, with higher concentrations in the upper layers. The retention time of naftifine in the skin was studied on the forearms of several human subjects with healthy forearm skin. The 3H-labeled 1% naftifine cream was applied and detected in the epidermis 5–10 days after the application with concentrations 3–5 times higher than the minimum inhibitory concentration (MIC) for *Trichophyton mentagrophytes*. Hence, a single application of naftifine a day is sufficient for the treatment of dermatophytic infections.[4]

In animal studies, naftifine was found to be entirely metabolized in the body and excreted in bile and urine. Naftifine is the active compound and none of its metabolites possesses antifungal activity.[1]

When 1% naftifine cream is applied once daily, 6% of the drug is absorbed systemically which has a half-life of 5–6 hours.[5]

Topical Formulations

Naftifine is available in three different formulations: 1% cream, 1% gel and 1% solution.

Uses

Naftifine is used in the treatment of fungal infections of the skin, hair and nails. It is active against *Trichophyton*, *Microsporum*, *Epidermophyton*, *Malassezia* and *Candida* species having the advantage of its anti-inflammatory property in addition to its fungicidal activity. It is, thus, used in the topical treatment of dermatophytic infections such as tinea corporis, tinea pedis and tinea cruris. It is also used for pityriasis versicolor and candidiasis.

One percent naftifine in its various formulations should be applied once daily uniformly as a thin film on the lesion as well as on 1 inch of the surrounding apparently normal skin.[1]

Side Effects

Side effects to naftifine are few and tolerable and include mild erythema and burning on application in a few subjects. There are scattered reports of allergic contact dermatitis to naftifine. Cross-sensitization and cross-reactivity with terbinafine can be an issue in these patients.[6]

Contraindications

Naftifine is a pregnancy category B drug. The package insert of the drug states that animal studies with naftifine concentrations 12–150 times the recommended topical use revealed no fetal harm. Limited application is probably safe although no human studies are available.[7]

Studies

Table 1 summarizes the studies conducted in various superficial fungal infections with naftifine.

Table 1: Studies Conducted in Various Superficial Fungal Infections with Naftifine*					
Condition treated	Number of subjects	Treatment regimen	Clinical cure (CC)	Mycological cure (MC)	Follow-up
Inflammatory tinea pedis, corporis, cruris[8]	63 vs. 59	1% naftifine cream once daily vs. miconazole/ hydrocortisone cream daily for 4 weeks			At 8 weeks: 95.2% vs. 44.1%
Tinea pedis[9]	99 enrolled, 90 analyzed	1% naftifine gel once daily vs. 1% terbinafine cream once daily vs. 1% oxiconazole cream once daily for 2 weeks	At 2 weeks 42.4% vs. 27.6% vs. 17.9%	At 2 weeks 33.3% vs. 34.5% vs. 21.4%	At 6 weeks, CC: 69.0% vs. 84.8% vs. 42.1% MC: 69.0% vs. 84.8% vs. 42.1% At 10 weeks, CC: 75% vs. 83.8% vs. 30.3% MC: 75% vs. 80.6% vs. 30.8%
Tinea cruris and corporis[10]	70	1% naftifine cream once daily for 4 weeks vs. vehicle once daily for 4 weeks			2 weeks post-treatment: MC 79% vs. 31%
Distal sub-ungual onychomy-cosis[11]	10	1% naftifine gel twice daily for 6 months	8/10 (80%)	8/10 (80%)	
Tinea corporis and cruris[12]	81 at onset of study, analysis of 62 patients	Naftifine 1% cream twice daily vs. vehicle cream twice daily		28/34 in naftifine group 9/28 in vehicle group	
Tinea pedis[13]	709	2% naftifine for 2 weeks (235) vs. vehicle (118) vs. 1% naftifine for 4 weeks (237) vs. vehicle (119)			At 6 weeks 67% MC, 22% CC in naftifine 2% group. Vehicle group 21% MC and 20% CC. MC and CC rates in both naftifine groups increased from weeks 2–6

Continued

Continued

Table 1: Studies Conducted in Various Superficial Fungal Infections with Naftifine*

Condition treated	Number of subjects	Treatment regimen	Clinical cure (CC)	Mycological cure (MC)	Follow-up
Tinea cruris[14]	344 enrolled. Analysis for 146 who had positive KOH and culture hence analyzed	2% naftifine cream once daily for 14 days vs. vehicle once daily for 14 days			At 4 weeks, 25% naftifine treated subjects had complete cure vs. 3% of vehicle treated subjects. 72% MC in naftifine group vs. 16% in vehicle group
Pediatric tinea corporis[15]	116 vs. 115	2% naftifine cream once daily for 2 weeks vs. vehicle once daily for 2 weeks. Analysis I 181 subjects with positive culture			Analysis in 181 subjects with positive culture. Statistically significant differences in CC and MC rates at week 3
Tinea versicolor[16]	10	1% naftifine gel twice daily for 2 weeks	1/10 KOH negative at 2 weeks		At 4 weeks, 5/10 (50%) negative Clinical symptom severity score 477 at baseline to 2.6 at week 4 and 2.7 at week 8 (scored from 0–9 with 0 = absent and 9 = worst)
Seborrheic dermatitis[17]	9	1% naftifine gel twice daily for 4 weeks			8/9 (89%) subjects reported improvement in symptoms at end of 4 weeks and 6 weeks. Erythema 38% less from baseline at 4 weeks, scaling 50% less at 4 and 6 weeks, itching reduced in 56% of subjects

*Only studies carried out in the last three decades are presented.

TERBINAFINE

Terbinafine, a synthetic allylamine antifungal agent is available orally and topically. This article focuses on topical terbinafine.

Chemistry

Terbinafine was designed by structurally modifying the allylamine molecule via addition of a benzene ring and triple bond (acetylene group) as well as a branched side chain.[18] The resultant compound, terbinafine was 10–100 times more potent than naftifine in vitro with markedly improved antifungal activity. Chemically terbinafine is E-N-(6,6-dimethyl-2-hepten-4-ynyl)-N-methyl-1-naphthalene-methanamine hydrochloride (Figure 3).

Mechanism of Action

Antifungal Activity

Terbinafine is the prototype allylamine which acts by inhibiting squalene epoxidase in a fashion similar to naftifine. The resultant lack of ergosterol downstream leads to fungistasis and accumulation of squalene with its subsequent deterrent intracellular effects leads to fungal cell death.

Terbinafine has a broad-spectrum of antifungal activity. It is chiefly fungicidal against dermatophytes, *Malassezia* species, molds and certain *Candida* species such as *C. parapsilosis;* terbinafine is fungistatic against *Candida albicans.*[18]

Pharmacokinetics

Terbinafine is a highly lipophilic drug with high affinity to the stratum corneum. It takes the transdermal route to reach its site of action. When 1% terbinafine cream is applied, it gets absorbed and binds to the lipophilic keratinocytes.[19] The cream is also found in high concentrations in the deepest part of the hair follicle. Less than 5% of 1% terbinafine cream gets absorbed into the system.

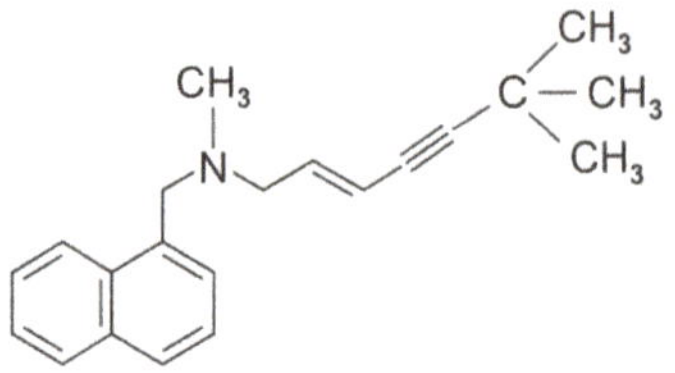

Figure 3: Chemical structure of terbinafine.

Formulations

Topical terbinafine is available as 1% cream, 1% gel and 1% spray.

Uses

Topical terbinafine is effective for the treatment of tinea corporis, tinea cruris, candidiasis and pityriasis versicolor. Topical terbinafine is applied twice daily for 2–4 weeks as shown in various studies (Table 2).

Table 2: Studies Conducted in Various Superficial Fungal Infections Treated with Terbinafine					
Intervention	Number of subjects	Clinical cure	Mycological cure	Complete cure	Follow-up
Budimulja et al.					
1% terbinafine cream vs. placebo once daily for 1 week in tinea cruris/corporis[21]	Total recruited 120; analysis for 57 vs. 60		53/57 (93%) in terbinafine group vs. 11/60 (18%) in placebo		
Cordero et al.					
1% terbinafine cream vs. placebo once daily for 1 week in tinea cruris/corporis[22]	Total recruited 74; analysis for 70 patients		27/29 in terbinafine group vs. 5/16 in placebo group	NA	NA
Lebwohl et al.					
1% terbinafine lotion vs. 1% vehicle[23]	66 recruited; 39 analyzed 20% drop out rate	17/23 vs. 2/16	21/23 vs. 10/16	NA	NA
van Heerden et al.					
1% terbinafine gel vs. vehicle gel once daily for 1 week in tinea corporis[24]	83 analysis for 60 patients	16/27 vs. 4/30	20/27 vs. 5/33	NA	NA
Vermeer et al.					
Terbinafine 1% solution vs. placebo twice daily for 1 week for pityriasis versicolor[25]	76 34	55 (72%) 9 (26%)	At 8 weeks 62 (81%) 14 (41%)	47% vs. 29%	

Continued

Continued

Table 2: Studies Conducted in Various Superficial Fungal Infections Treated with Terbinafine					
Intervention	Number of subjects	Clinical cure	Mycological cure	Complete cure	Follow-up
Savin et al.					
Terbinafine 1% solution vs. vehicle twice daily for 7 days for pityriasis versicolor[26]	96 46	45 (47%) 14 (30%)	At 1 week 57 (59%) 26 (56%)		At 8 weeks, clinical cure rate 81% vs. 31%, mycological cure rate 82% vs. 32%
Budimulja et al.					
A. Terbinafine 1% solution vs. vehicle twice daily for 1 week B. Terbinafine 1% solution once daily for1 week for pityriasis versicolor[27]	192 vs. 96 50 vs. 50		At 2 weeks, 108 (56%) vs. 34 (35%) in group		Mycological cure at 8 weeks: 123 (64%) vs. 32 (33%) in group A and 25 (50%) vs. 14 (28%) in group B
Faergemann et al.					
Terbinafine 1% emulsion gel vs. placebo gel once daily for 1 week for pityriasis versicolor[28]	31 vs. 30			11/29 (39%) vs. 7/29 (24%)	At 8 weeks, 21/28 (75%) vs. 4/29 (14%) remained completely cured

Side Effects

Terbinafine is well-tolerated in its topical form with few side effects rarely.

Terbinafine is a pregnancy category B drug. A prospective study in 54 pregnant women (44% in first trimester) who had used terbinafine (26 oral) did not reveal any teratogenicity.[20] Due to paucity of human data, safer alternatives such as clotrimazole and miconazole should be preferred.[7]

BUTENAFINE

Butenafine is a newer topical antifungal belonging to the benzylamine class of antifungals. It was first approved in Japan in 1992 and later on in the United States of America in 1997.

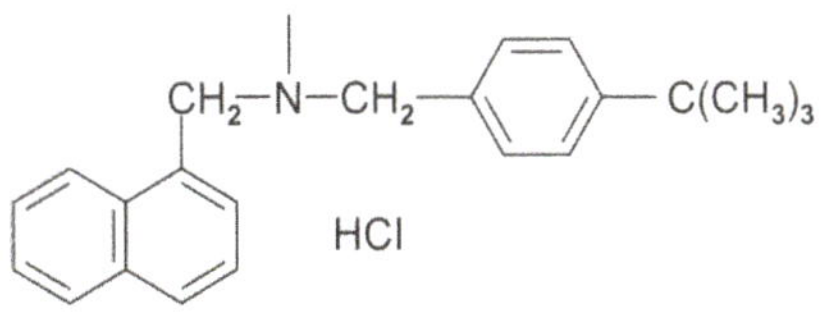

Figure 4: Chemical structure of butenafine.

Chemistry

Butenafine is structurally similar to the allylamine antifungals with the exception of a butylbenzyl group that replaces the allylamine group. This structural alteration produced a compound with enhanced antimycotic activity compared to terbinafine and naftifine. Butenafine is N-4-tert-butylbenzyl-N-methyl-1-naphthalenemethylamine hydrochloride (Figure 4).

Mechanism of Action

Butenafine acts in a way similar to the allylamines via inhibition of squalene epoxidase with resultant deprivement of products required for fungal cell membrane synthesis. It thus, has fungicidal effects just like the allylamines. In addition to this property, it also has an anti-inflammatory activity.

Pharmacokinetics

Butenafine penetrates the epidermis and this effect was studied in guinea pigs using C^{14}-labeled 0.2 mL of 1% butenafine cream. In this experiment, high concentrations of butenafine were found throughout the epidermis with the highest concentration in the stratum corneum. Very low concentrations were found in the sebaceous glands and hair follicles implicating poor penetration into these areas.[29,30]

The MIC of butenafine against *T. mentagrophytes* and *Microsporum canis* was 4–65 times lower than that of clotrimazole, naftifine, tolnaftate, and bifonazole and the minimum fungicidal concentration was 4–130 times lower than the above drugs.

Butenafine easily gets incorporated into membrane phospholipids in keratinocytes, from where it is released slowly and acts on infected cells, hence, explaining its long duration of fungicidal activity. Systemic absorption is negligible.

Formulations

Butenafine is available as 1% cream.

Uses

It was first licensed for usage for the treatment of tinea corporis, tinea cruris and tinea pedis in Japan in 1992. Subsequently, it received licensure in the United States.

It has extensively been studied in Japan and the United States for use in tinea corporis, tinea cruris and tinea pedis. It is also used in the treatment of pityriasis versicolor, tinea nigra and seborrheic dermatitis.

Side Effects

Butenafine is well-tolerated. Few patients develop burning or stinging after application that does not warrant withdrawal.

Butenafine is a pregnancy category C drug. Although human studies are lacking, animal studies did not show any mutagenic effects, hence, use for a limited time and area is probably safe in pregnancy (Table 3).

Table 3: Studies Conducted in Various Superficial Fungal Infections with Butenafine					
Intervention	Number of subjects	Clinical cure (CC)	Mycologic cure (MC)	Complete cure (CoC)	Follow-up
Savin et al.					
A. 1% butenafine cream for 7 days in tinea pedis B. Vehicle once daily for 7 days in tinea pedis[31]	132 vs. 139	At 8 days, 6% (A) vs. 1% (B) At 14 days, 17% (A) vs. 9% (B) At 5 weeks, 40% (A) vs. 9% (B)	At 8 days, 43% (A) vs. 25% (B)	At 14 days, 4% (A) vs. 0% (B) At 5 weeks 20% (A) vs. 1% (B)	At 14 days, MC 61% (A) vs. 35% (B) At 5 weeks, MC 74% (A) vs. 22% (B)
Tschen et al.					
A. 1% butenafiine cream once daily for 4 weeks in tinea pedis B. Vehicle once daily for 4 weeks in tinea pedis[32]	40 40		At 4 weeks, 40% (A) vs. 20% (B)		At 4 weeks, MC rate 88% (A) vs. 45% (B) At 8 weeks, MC 88% (A) vs. 33% (B)

Continued

Continued

Table 3: Studies Conducted in Various Superficial Fungal Infections with Butenafine

Intervention	Number of subjects	Clinical cure (CC)	Mycologic cure (MC)	Complete cure (CoC)	Follow-up
Lesher et al.					
A. 1% butenafine cream once daily for 2 weeks in tinea cruris B. Vehicle once daily for 2 weeks in tinea cruris[33]	37 39		At 7 days, 66% (A) vs. 13% (B)	At day 14, overall cure rates 31% (A) vs. 8% (B)	At day 42, MC 81% (A) vs. 13% (B). At day 42, overall cure rate 62% (A) vs. 4% (B)
Greer et al.					
A. 1% butenafine cream once daily for 2 weeks in tinea corporis B. Vehicle once daily for 2 weeks[34]	42 36		At day 14, 88% (A) vs. 28% (B)	At day 14, 31% (A) vs. 3% (B)	At day 42, MC 88% (A) vs. 17% (B) overall cure rate 67% (A) vs. 14% (B)

CONCLUSION

The allylamines and benzylamine antifungals are a unique class of agents with fungicidal, anti-inflammatory, and prolonged post-treatment residual antifungal activity. They are preferred as first-line topical agents in dermatophytic fungal infections and are also a useful armamentarium for candidiasis, pityriasis versicolor and tinea nigra.

REFERENCES

1. Mühlbacher JM. Naftifine: a topical allylamine antifungal agent. *Clin Dermatol.* 1992;9(4):479-85.
2. Evans EG, James IG, Seaman RA, Richardson MD. Does naftifine have anti-inflammatory properties? A double-blind comparative study with 1% clotrimazole/1% hydrocortisone in clinically diagnosed fungal infection of the skin. *Br J Dermatol.* 1993;129(4):437-42.
3. Stuttgen G. Biopharmaceutical aspects of topically applied antifungal treatment. *Mykosen.* 1987;30(Suppl 1):7-14.
4. Czok R. Preclinical evaluation of Exoderil (naftifine). Part II. Mechanism of action, absorption, metabolism and excretion. *Mykosen.* 1987;30(Suppl 1):28-31.

5. Gupta AK. Ryder JE, Cooper EA. Natftifine: a review. *J Cut Med Surg*. 2008;12(2):51-8.

6. Corazza M, Lauriola MM, Virgili A. Allergic contact dermatitis to naftifine. *Contact Dermatitis*. 2005;53(5):302-3.

7. Patel VM, Schwartz RA, Lambert WC. Topical antiviral and antifungal medications in pregnancy: a review of safety profiles. *J Eur Acad Dermatol Venereol*. 2017;31(9):1440-6.

8. Nada M, Hanafi S, al-Omari H, et al. Naftifine versus miconazole/hydrocortisone in inflammatory dermatophyte infections. *Int J Dermatol*. 1994;33(8):570-2.

9. Ablon G, Rosen T, Spedale J. Comparative efficacy of naftifine, oxiconazole, and terbinafine in short-term treatment of tinea pedis. *Int J Dermatol*. 1996;35(8):591-3.

10. Jordon RE, Rapini RP, Rex IH Jr, Katz HI, Hickman JG, Bard JW, et al. Once-daily naftifine cream 1% in the treatment of tinea cruris and tinea corporis. *Int J Dermatol*. 1990;29(6):441-2.

11. Meyerson MS, Scher RK, Hochman LG, et al. Open-label study of the safety and efficacy of naftifine hydrochloride 1% gel in patients with distal subungual onychomycosis of the fingers. *Cutis*. 1993;51(3):205-7.

12. Dobson RL, Bagatell FK, Hickman JG, et al. Naftifine 1% cream in the treatment of tinea cruris and tinea corporis. *Drug Invest*. 1993;3:57-9.

13. Parish LC, Parish JL, Routh HB, et al. A randomized, double-blind, vehicle-controlled efficacy and safety study of naftifine 2% cream in the treatment of tinea pedis. *J Drugs Dermatol*. 2011;10(11):1282-8.

14. Parish LC, Parish JL, Routh HB, et al. A double-blind, randomized, vehicle-controlled study evaluating the efficacy and safety of naftifine 2% cream in tinea cruris. *J Drugs Dermatol*. 2011;10(10):1142-7.

15. Gold M, Dhawan S, Verma A, Kuligowski M, Dobrowski D. Efficacy and safety of naftifine HCl cream 2% in the treatment of pediatric subjects with tinea corporis. *J Drugs Dermatol*. 2016;15(6):743-8.

16. Gold MH, Bridges T, Avakian E, et al. An open-label study of naftifine hydrochloride 1% gel in the treatment of tinea versicolor. *Skinmed*. 2011;9(5):283-6.

17. Gold MH, Bridges T, Avakian EV, et al. An open-label pilot study of naftifine 1% gel in the treatment of seborrheic dermatitis of the scalp. *J Drugs Dermatol*. 2012;11(4):514-8.

18. Shear NH, Villars VV, Marsolais C. Terbinafine: an oral and topical antifungal agent. *Clin Dermatol*. 1992;9(4):487-95.

19. Faergemann J, Zehender H, Jones T, Maibach I. Terbinafine levels in serum, stratum corneum, dermis-epidermis (without stratum corneum), hair, sebum and eccrine sweat. *Acta Derm Venereol*. 1990;71(4):322-6.

20. Sarkar M, Rowland K, Koren G. Pregnancy outcomes following gestational exposure to terbinafine: a prospective comparative study. *Clin Mol Teratol*. 2003;67(5):390.

21. Budimulja U, Bramono K, Urip KS, et al. Once-daily treatment with terbinafine 1% cream (Lamisil) for one week is effective in the treatment of tinea corporis and cruris. A placebo-controlled study. *Mycoses*. 2001;44(7-8):300-6.

22. Cordero C, de la Rosa I, Espinosa Z, Rojas RF, Zaias N. Short-term therapy of tinea cruris/corporis with topical terbinafine. *J Dermatol Treat*. 1992;3(Suppl 1):23-4.

23. Lebwohl M, Elewski B, Eisen D, Savin RC. Efficacy and safety of terbinafine 1% solution in the treatment of interdigital tinea pedis and tinea corporis or tinea cruris. *Cutis*. 2001;67(3):261-6.

24. van Heerden JS, Vismer HF. Tinea corporis/cruris: new treatment options. *Dermatology*. 1997;194(Suppl 1):14-8.

25. Vermeer BJ, Staats CC. The efficacy of a topical application of terbinafine 1% solution in subjects with pityriasis versicolor: a placebo-controlled study. *Dermatology*. 1997;194(Suppl):122-4.

26. Savin R, Eisen D, Fradin MS, Lebwohl M. Tinea versicolor treated with terbinafine 1% solution. *Int J Dermatol*. 1999;31(11):863-5.

27. Budimulja U, Paul C. One-week terbinafine 1% solution in pityriasis versicolor: twice-daily application is more effective than once-daily. *J Dermatolog Treat*. 2002;13(1):39-40.

28. Faergemann J, Hersle K, Nordin P. Pityriasis versicolor: clinical experience with Lamisil cream and Lamisil DermGel. *Dermatology*. 1997;194(Suppl 1):19-21.

29. McNeely W, Spencer CM. Butenafine. *Drugs*. 1998;55(3):405-13.

30. Singal A. Butenafine and superficial mycoses: current status. *Expert Opin Drug Metab Toxicol.* 2008;4(7):999-1005.

31. Savin R, De Villez RL, Elewski B, et al. One-week therapy with twice-daily butenafine 1% cream versus vehicle in the treatment of tinea pedis: a multicenter, double-blind trial. *J Am Acad Dermatol.* 1997;36(2 Pt 1):S15-9.

32. Tschen E, Elewski B, Gorsulowsky DC, Pariser DM. Treatment of interdigital tinea pedis with a 4-week once-daily regimen of butenafine hydrochloride 1% cream. *J Am Acad Dermatol.* 1997;36(2 Pt 1):S9-14.

33. Lesher JL Jr, Babel DE, Stewart DM, et al. Butenafine 1% cream in the treatment of tinea cruris: a multicenter, vehicle-controlled, double-blind trial. *J Am Acad Dermatol.* 1997;36(2 Pt 1):S20-4.

34. Greer DL, Weiss J, Rodriguez DA, Hebert AA, Swinehart JM. A randomized trial to assess once-daily topical treatment of tinea corporis with butenafine, a new antifungal agent. *J Am Acad Dermatol.* 1997;37(2 Pt 1):231-5.

World Clin Dermatol. 2019;5(1):82-100.

Topical Azole Antifungals

*Mala Bhalla MD, Priyanka Sharma MD

Department of Dermatology, Venereology and Leprosy,
Government Medical College and Hospital, Chandigarh, Punjab, India

ABSTRACT

Topical azoles are one of the commonly used antifungal agents used for the treatment of superficial fungal infections. These play an important role as first-line therapy in localized uncomplicated superficial mycoses and as adjuvant for widespread infections. Various newer topical azoles with improved pharmacokinetics have also been introduced in the recent years. This article discusses the details of topical azoles and their role in the management of various cutaneous superficial mycoses.

INTRODUCTION

Superficial cutaneous mycoses represent one of the most common dermatological diseases affecting 20–25% of the world's population.[1] Treatment of these infections depends upon the extent, site and severity of infection. While the localized and uncomplicated superficial fungal infections can be managed with topical antifungals alone, oral antifungals form the cornerstone for the treatment of widespread and complicated infections. The topical antifungals play an important role as adjuvant to systemic therapy owing to their better pharmacokinetics, and hence, better clearance of infection when combined with systemic agents. Since the topical antifungals have limited percutaneous absorption, the risk of drug interactions and systemic adverse effects are of less concern. Thus, topical agents are safer and may be preferred over systemic counterparts in special situations like pregnancy, lactation, infancy, and systemic comorbidities like severe hepatic and renal disorders.

Based on their mechanism of action, topical antifungals can be divided into: (1) azoles, (2) allylamines/benzylamines, (3) polyenes, and (4) miscellaneous group

---

*Corresponding author
Email: malabhalla@yahoo.co.in

including ciclopirox olamine, selenium sulfide, zinc pyrithione, morpholines, oxaboroles and tolnaftate.

TOPICAL AZOLES

Topical azoles are broad-spectrum antifungal agents which have a basic structural unit consisting of a five-membered aromatic azole ring. Depending upon the number of nitrogen molecules in the azole ring, they are further divided into two subgroups—imidazoles and triazoles. The imidazoles have two while triazoles have three nitrogen molecules attached to the azole ring (Figure 1). Variation in

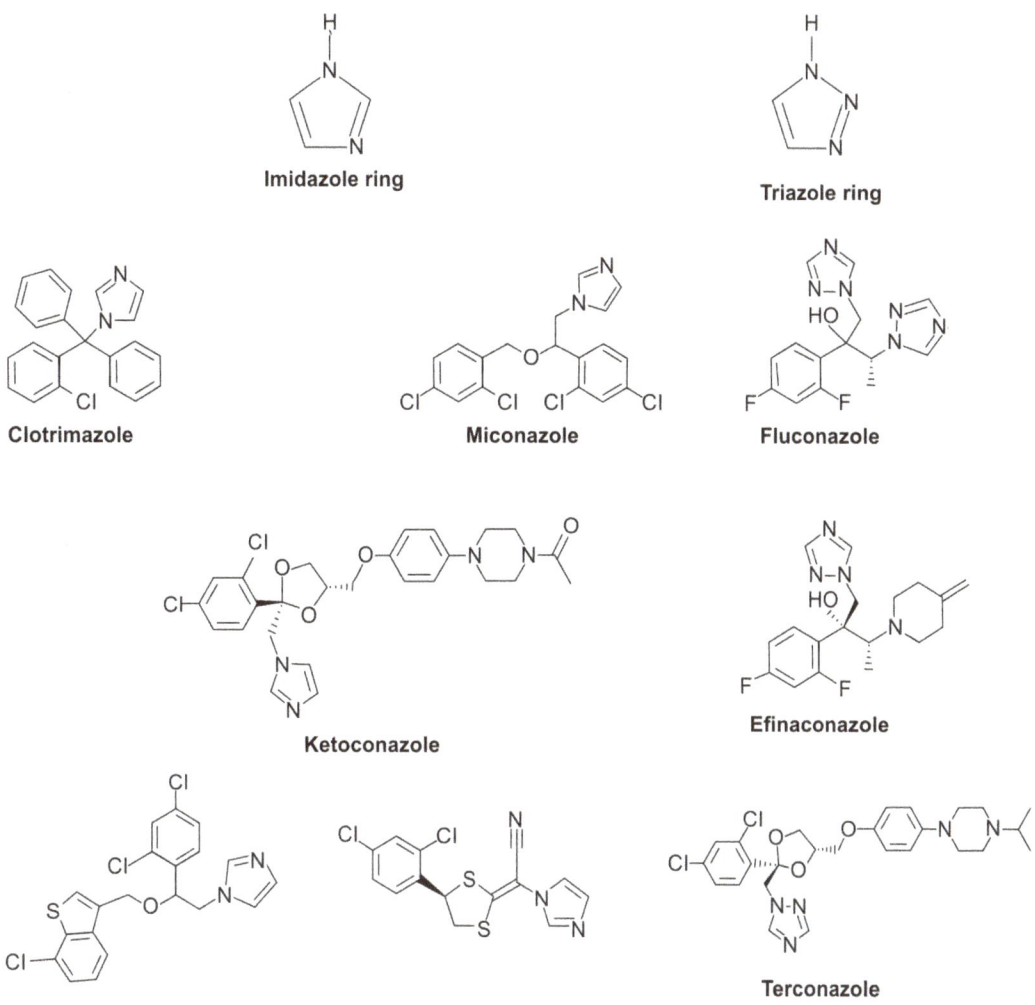

Figure 1: Chemical structure of common topical azoles.

molecular weight, side-chain structure of azole ring, and water solubility determine the pharmacokinetic characteristics and antifungal activity of individual drugs.

Currently available topical imidazole compounds include clotrimazole, miconazole, ketoconazole, econazole, bifonazole, oxiconazole, tioconazole and lanoconazole with some newer introductions such as sertaconazole, luliconazole and eberconazole. The topical triazoles include fluconazole, efinaconazole and terconazole. Further, these are available in different concentrations and compounded into conventional as well as newer vehicles which affect the drug penetration through stratum corneum and efficacy of the parent compound (Table 1).

Table 1: List of Topical Azoles and their Formulations			
Subgroup	Drugs	Available concentration and conventional formulations	Frequency of application[2]
Imidazoles	Clotrimazole	1% cream, solution/lotion, powder, mouth paint, oral troche, tincture, vaginal cream and suppositories	Twice daily; 4–6 weeks
	Ketoconazole	2% cream, gel, lotion, foam, vaginal cream and suppositories, 1% and 2% shampoo	Once daily; 2–4 weeks
	Miconazole	2% cream, oral gel, lotion, powder, spray, vaginal suppositories	Twice daily; 4–6 weeks Suppositories—Once daily for 3 days
	Econazole	1% cream, foam, spray, powder, vaginal cream and suppositories	Once/twice daily; 2–4 weeks
	Bifonazole	1% cream, gel, solution, powder	Once daily; 4 weeks
	Oxiconazole	1% cream, lotion	Once daily; 4–6 weeks
	Tioconazole	1% and 2% cream, gel, 6.5% vaginal ointment, vaginal pessaries, 28% nail solution	Cream/lotion—Twice daily; 4 weeks Nail solution—Twice daily; 6–12 months
	Eberconazole	1% cream, foam, lotion	Twice daily; 2–4 weeks
	Sertaconazole	2% cream, lotion, shampoo	Twice daily; 4 weeks
	Luliconazole	1% cream, lotion	Once daily; 2–4 weeks
	Sulconazole	1% cream, lotion	Once/twice daily; 2–4 weeks
	Fenticonazole	2% cream, lotion, vaginal capsules	Twice daily; 4 weeks
Triazoles	Fluconazole	0.5% gel	Twice daily; 4 weeks
	Efinaconazole	10% nail solution	48 weeks for toenail onychomycosis
	Terconazole	0.4% and 0.8% vaginal cream, vaginal suppository	Once daily for 7 or 3 consecutive days

HISTORY

First azole compound, benzimidazole and its substituted derivates were reported in 1944 by Woolley while studying biotin deficiency in animals and microbes. Benzimidazole, a compound derived from biotin was found to have inhibitory effects on yeasts. Later, in 1969, clotrimazole, miconazole and econazole were developed and introduced as new broad-spectrum imidazole compounds. Ketoconazole, a broad-spectrum imidazole, was introduced in 1977. Subsequently, newer azole compounds were developed including sulconazole, oxiconazole, bifonazole, and tioconazole.[3] Sertaconazole, eberconazole, and luliconazole represent even more recent antifungal azoles with improved pharmacokinetics and broader-spectrum of antifungal activity.

MECHANISM OF ACTION

The azoles exert fungistatic effect by inhibiting the pathway of fungal cell wall ergosterol biosynthesis which serves as a bioregulator of membrane fluidity and integrity of fungal cells. These drugs inhibit the cytochrome P450-dependent enzyme, lanosterol 14α-demethylase which catalyzes the conversion of lanosterol into ergosterol. Due to the depletion of ergosterol and accumulation of intracellular 14α-methylsterols, there is alteration in membrane rigidity and permeability, ultimately leading to fungal cell death.[4] Certain azoles such as sertaconazole, luliconazole and eberconazole exhibit anti-inflammatory effect which is thought to be mediated via inhibition of arachadonic acid pathway.[5]

SPECTRUM OF ANTIFUNGAL ACTIVITY

Azoles have a wide spectrum of activity against various fungal pathogens which varies with each compound. They are primarily active against dermatophytes, i.e. most of the *Trichophyton*, *Microsporum* and *Epidermophyton* species, *Candida albicans*, *Candida neoformans*, *Candida glabrata*, dimorphic fungi, *Aspergillus* and *Fusarium* species. Individual variation in the antifungal activity may be attributable to differences in 14α-demethylase enzyme inhibition and secondary targets of drugs.[6] Certain azoles such as clotrimazole, econazole, miconazole and sertaconazole possess in vitro activity against gram-positive bacteria.[7]

IMIDAZOLE DERIVATIVES

Clotrimazole

Pharmacology

Clotrimazole is one of the first synthetic imidazole antifungals, synthesized in 1969.[8] The percutaneous absorption of clotrimazole is negligible; small amounts absorbed are metabolized in the liver and excreted in the bile. About 5–10% fraction is absorbed following vaginal application of clotrimazole.

Spectrum of Activity

Clotrimazole shows in vitro antifungal activity against most dermatophytes, *Candida* species, *Malassezia furfur*, and few strains of gram-positive bacteria. At higher concentrations, clotrimazole has demonstrated inhibitory effect on *Trichomonas* species.[9] Although, in vitro antifungal activity of clotrimazole against filamentous and dimorphic fungi is comparable to that of other antifungal agents such as griseofulvin, amphotericin B and nystatin, the use of clotrimazole is limited to topical application because of undesirable side effects following oral intake.[10]

Clinical Use

It is available in various forms such as cream, lotion, solution, powder, oral troche and vaginal pessaries. The recommended dose is twice daily application for the treatment of superficial cutaneous as well as vaginal fungal infections such as dermatophytosis, pityriasis versicolor, cutaneous and vaginal candidiasis. Clotrimazole vaginal tablet/pessaries of various strengths (100 mg, 200 mg, and 600 mg) have been formulated and proven efficacious in even once daily dose for the treatment of vulvovaginal candidiasis.[11] Clotrimazole oral troches (10 mg) and solution are also available for the treatment of oral candidiasis.[12]

Miconazole

Pharmacology

Miconazole is a synthetic β-substituted 1-phenethyl imidazole which was introduced in 1969 (Figure 1). It is very slightly soluble in water and most organic solvents. While its penetration of stratum corneum is good, the percutaneous absorption is minimal (i.e. <1%). Like other azoles, it also inhibits lanosterol 14α-demethylase enzyme which interferes with fungal cell wall ergosterol synthesis, but at high concentrations, it may exert cell membrane damaging effect leading to fungal cell death.[13]

Spectrum of Activity

Miconazole shows in vitro activity against common dermatophytes, especially *Trichophyton rubrum*, *Trichophyton mentagrophytes* and *Epidermophyton floccosum*, *C. albicans*, *non-albicans Candida* species, *Malassezia* species, *Aspergillus fumigatus* and *Sporothrix schenckii*. Mycetoma-causing agents such as *Madurella mycetomatis*, *Streptomyces* and *Nocardia* species also show sensitivity to miconazole.[13]

Clinical Use

Miconazole is available in the form of 2% cream, oral gel, lotion, powder and spray. It is indicated in the treatment of dermatophytic infections, pityriasis versicolor, cutaneous and vaginal candidiasis. Miconazole vaginal suppositories in the dose of 100 mg, 200 mg and 1,200 mg are effective in vaginal candidiasis when used for 7 days, 3 days and 1 day, respectively. It also exhibits some activity against few gram-positive bacteria such as group A β-hemolytic streptococci, staphylococci, and corynebacteria. Miconazole has been found effective in erythrasma, impetigo and ecthyma.[14]

Ketoconazole

Pharmacology

Ketoconazole is a synthetic water-soluble imidazole broad-spectrum antifungal, synthesized and developed in 1977 by Janssen Pharmaceutical.[15] Percutaneous absorption of topical 2% ketoconazole is very poor and it is minimally absorbed from vagina.[16]

Spectrum of Activity

Ketoconazole is a broad-spectrum antifungal which exhibits activity against most dermatophytes of all three genera, *Candida* species, *Pityrosporum ovale*, molds, *Rhodotorula* species and *Saccharomyces cerevisiae*.[15]

Clinical Use

Ketoconazole is available as 2% cream, gel, foam, and 1% and 2% shampoo formulations. It has been used in the treatment of tinea pedis, tinea cruris and tinea corporis.[17] Once daily application of ketoconazole for duration of 4 weeks has shown excellent results in dermatophytosis. It has also been used effectively in the treatment of pityriasis versicolor, considering *P. ovale* as one of the causative agent.[18] Ketoconazole lotion, shampoo and novel foam formulations have been found to be efficacious in seborrheic dermatitis. About 1% shampoo formulation of ketoconazole is approved for over-the-counter use in the management of seborrheic dermatitis.[19] Ketoconazole cream and vaginal suppositories are also effective in the treatment of cutaneous candidiasis.[20]

Econazole

Pharmacology

Econazole is a deschloro derivative of miconazole, first synthesized in 1969. It shows poor systemic absorption following topical application and is only minimally recovered in the urine and feces. When applied topically, approximately 90% of the drug remains on the skin surface. About 3–7% fraction is absorbed following vaginal application of econazole.[21]

Spectrum of Activity

Econazole shows in vitro antifungal activity against most strains of *Trichophyton*, *Microsporum* and *Epidermophyton* species, *C. albicans*, *Candida tropicalis*, actinomycetes, *P. ovale* and molds. In addition, it also inhibits some gram-positive and gram-negative bacilli and cocci; the minimum inhibitory concentration (MIC) being similar to those for yeasts.[21] It does not appear to affect gram-negative bacteria.

Clinical Use

It is available as 1% econazole nitrate cream and foam formulation; latter being easier to apply and more esthetically pleasing than cream. Econazole has been approved for the treatment of tinea cruris, tinea corporis, tinea pedis, pityriasis versicolor and cutaneous candidiasis; the recommended dosage is twice daily application for several weeks.[22] It has been used effectively for the treatment of interdigital toe web bacterial infections.[23] In patients with otomycosis, usually due to *Candida* or *Aspergillus* species, econazole 1% solution for 1–3 weeks has been proved to be curative.[24] Econazole vaginal cream and suppositories have been used in the management of vaginal candidiasis; two dosage regimens have been used—a 3-day therapy using a 150 mg vaginal suppository daily, or 2 weeks therapy using a 50 mg suppository once daily.[21]

Sertaconazole

Pharmacology

Sertaconazole is a novel imidazole drug with improved pharmacokinetics due to its unique chemical structure. It contains a benzothiophene ring which mimics tryptophan and increases the drugs ability to form pores in the fungal cell membrane.[25] Additionally, the lipophilic benzothiophene ring renders the drug more lipophilic than other azoles, enabling the dermal reservoir effect, and thus, attaining the fungicidal concentration in skin layers.[26] Besides its indirect inhibitory effect on fungal cell wall ergosterol biosynthesis, at higher concentrations, it binds directly to nonsterol lipids in the fungal cell wall, which leads to direct cell membrane damage.[27] Sertaconazole also possesses anti-inflammatory and anti-pruritic properties which has been evaluated in both in vitro and animal studies.[28]

Spectrum of Activity

Sertaconazole inhibits most dermatophytes of the *Trichophyton, Epidermophyton,* and *Microsporum* genera, *Candida* species, *Scedosporium, Scopulariopsis, Cryptococcus* species, *Aspergillus* and various opportunistic filamentous fungi. It exhibits in vitro fungicidal activity against limited number of *Candida* species and *T. mentagrophytes.*[27] Sertaconazole also shows antimicrobial activity against gram-positive bacteria from *Staphylococcus* and *Streptococcus* genera and protozoa such as *Trichomonas vaginalis.*[25]

Clinical Use

It is available as 2% sertaconazole nitrate cream, gel, lotion, powder and shampoo formulations. Sertaconazole is the Food and Drug Administration (FDA)-approved for the treatment of tinea pedis caused by *T. rubrum, Trichophyton interdigitale* and *E. floccosum* in 12 years or older individuals. The recommended regimen for tinea pedis is once or twice daily application for 4 weeks. It is also efficacious in the treatment of other dermatophytosis, cutaneous candidiasis, pityriasis versicolor and seborrheic dermatitis of the scalp.[25]

Oxiconazole

Pharmacology

Oxiconazole nitrate is an acetophenone oxime derivative of the imidazole, first approved in the United States in 1989 for the treatment of human dermatophytosis.[29] Following rapid absorption of topical oxiconazole into the stratum corneum, it attains the maximum concentration in epidermis and dermis within 100 minutes. It has been demonstrated in animal studies that oxiconazole persists in horny layer of skin for up to 96 hours after a single application.[30] Because of its reservoir effect in epidermis and dermis, once daily dosing of oxiconazole is sufficient to eradicate the superficial fungi. Percutaneous absorption of topical oxiconazole is negligible with only <0.3% fraction recovered in the urine and none recovered in feces.[31]

Spectrum of Activity

Oxiconazole has a broad-spectrum of activity against most dermatophytes, *Trichosporon cutaneum*, *C. albicans* and *M. furfur*. It is also active against *Torulopsis glabrata*, *A. fumigatus* and *Cryptococcus neoformans* as well as gram-positive bacteria including *Corynebacterium minutissimum*.[29]

Clinical Use

Oxiconazole is commercially available as 1% cream and lotion form, the latter is preferred in cases of larger or hairy areas. It has been used effectively for the treatment of tinea pedis, tinea cruris, tinea corporis, cutaneous candidiasis and pityriasis versicolor. It has also proven efficacious in cases of erythrasma, owing to its inhibitory effect on corynebacteria.[32]

Luliconazole

Pharmacology

Luliconazole is a novel imidazole antifungal, developed and approved in Japan in 2005. It has an imidazole moiety incorporated into the ketone dithioacetate structure. This unique modification in its chemical structure results in higher potency and a wider spectrum of activity of luliconazole against various fungal pathogens. It is an optically active R-enantiomer of lanoconazole, with more potent antifungal activity than the latter.[33]

Spectrum of Activity

Luliconazole shows potent in vitro antifungal activity against most dermatophytes especially *Trichophyton* species, *C. albicans*, *M. furfur*, *Malassezia restricta* and *A. fumigatus*. The in vitro antifungal activity of luliconazole against Trichophyton spp. has been found to be the highest among other topical antifungal drugs.[34]

Clinical Use

Luliconazole is available as 1% cream and lotion form. Luliconazole 1% cream is indicated for the treatment of tinea cruris, tinea corporis and interdigital tinea pedis, in 18 years and older individuals.[33] The recommended dosage is once daily application for 1 week in tinea corporis and tinea cruris and for 2 weeks in tinea pedis. It has also been used effectively in the treatment of cutaneous candidiasis, pityriasis versicolor and seborrheic dermatitis.[35]

Bifonazole

Pharmacology

Bifonazole is a substituted imidazole compound with broad-spectrum of activity against fungal pathogens. Following topical application, it attains concentration in epidermis, higher than the MIC for most dermatophytes. Because of its potent antifungal activity and reservoir effect in the skin, bifonazole was the first topical antifungal agent to be used in a once daily regimen.[36]

Spectrum of Activity

In vitro susceptibility tests have demonstrated its potent and broad-spectrum of antifungal activity against dermatophytes, yeasts, molds and dimorphic fungi, usually at concentrations of less than 4 mg/L, which is similar to clotrimazole and miconazole.[37]

Clinical Use

It is available as 1% cream, gel, solution and powder forms. Bifonazole has been used effectively for treatment of superficial mycoses such as dermatophytoses, cutaneous candidiasis and pityriasis versicolor. In controlled comparative trials, the efficacy of once daily application of bifonazole has been found to be as efficacious as that of other topical imidazoles such as clotrimazole, econazole, miconazole and sulconazole, applied twice daily. The recommended regimen for the treatment of dermatomycoses is once daily for 2–4 weeks, although prolonged therapy is needed in cases of tinea pedis and manuum.[38]

Tioconazole

Pharmacology

Tioconazole is a synthetic 1-substituted imidazole antifungal agent with dual mode action that is indirect inhibition of sterol biosynthesis as well as direct cell membrane damage leading to leakage of cell contents. Following topical application of various formulations of tioconazole, it is minimally absorbed into the systemic circulation.[39]

Spectrum of Activity

Tioconazole is active against most dermatophytes, *Candida* species, *C. neoformans*, *T. glabrata*, *Aspergillus* species, chlamydia, *Gardnerella vaginalis*, *T. vaginalis* and gram-positive bacteria including *C. minutissimum*, various strains of *Streptococcus* and *Staphylococcus*. In vitro and animal studies have shown tioconazole to be more active than miconazole and clotrimazole.[40]

Clinical Use

It is available as 1% and 2% tioconazole hydrochloride cream/gel, 6.5% vaginal ointment, vaginal pessaries of 100 mg and 300 mg and 28% nail solution. Tioconazole has been proven to be efficacious in dermatophytosis, pityriasis versicolor, and cutaneous and vaginal candidiasis. Tioconazole vaginal pessaries are recommended in dosage of 100 mg once daily at bed time for 3, 6, or 14 days, or as 300 mg single bed time application.[41] About 28% tioconazole nail solution has been formulated for treatment of onychomycosis, with a recommended dose of twice daily application for prolonged duration of up to 12 months.[42]

Eberconazole

Pharmacology

Eberconazole is a novel imidazole antifungal agent known to have steroid synthesis inhibitory action. It was developed in Spain and launched in 2005. Following topical application, it is minimally absorbed systemically and its concentration remains undetected in human plasma and urine.[43] Depending upon its concentration, eberconazole has dual mode of action; at lower concentrations, it prevents fungal cell growth by inhibiting lanosterol 14α-demethylase whereas at high concentrations, it exerts fungicidal effect by causing the leakage of small intracellular molecules from the fungal cell leading to cell death. It also possesses anti-inflammatory property which is due to inhibition of 5-lipooxygenase and to a lesser extent of cyclooxygenase-2 mediated pathways of inflammation.[44]

Spectrum of Activity

Inhibitory effect of eberconazole has been demonstrated against most strains of dermatophyte genera, *Candida* species, *M. furfur* and few gram-positive bacteria in in vitro and animal studies, with similar or even higher efficacy than clotrimazole and ketoconazole against various strains of *Candida*, especially, triazole-resistant yeasts (*C. krusei* and *C. glabrata*) and fluconazole-resistant *C. albicans*.[43] In vitro activity of eberconazole has been found to be higher than miconazole, clotrimazole and ketoconazole against dermatophytic fungi.[45]

Clinical Use

It is available as 1% eberconazole nitrate cream, foam and lotion forms for use in cutaneous mycoses. It is effective in twice daily application for the treatment of dermatophytosis, pityriasis versicolor, cutaneous and vaginal candidiasis. In a double blind study, the efficacy and safety profile of eberconazole 1% cream was comparable to miconazole.[46] Also there is a novel formulation recently made available which is a non-alcoholic creamy Eberconazole lotion. This lotion could be specifically used and better suited for extensive tinea corporis wherein large and numerous lesions appear.

Sulconazole

Pharmacology

Sulconazole differs from the other azoles by having a sulfide (thiol) bond between constituent rings.[47] When applied topically, about 12% fraction of the drug is percutaneously absorbed. It may be detected in the stratum corneum for up to 96 hours after application.[48] Besides its indirect fungistatic effect on ergosterol biosynthesis, it exerts fungicidal effects by causing direct cell membrane damage.[49]

Spectrum of Activity

Sulconazole exhibits in vitro activity against dermatophytes, yeasts and molds, gram-positive bacteria such as *Staphylococcus aureus*, *Staphylococcus epidermidis*, *Streptococcus faecalis,* and certain gram-positive anaerobes including *Clostridium* species At higher concentrations, it shows fungicidal effects against *C. albicans* and *Candida pseudotropicalis.*[50]

Clinical Use

Sulconazole nitrate is available as 1% cream and solution form. It has been used effectively for the treatment of *Candida* infections, tinea cruris, tinea corporis, tinea pedis and pityriasis versicolor. The recommended dosage is twice daily application for 3–4 weeks. Sulconazole 1% cream has been found to be more efficacious than clotrimazole, econazole and miconazole.[49] Owing to its effect on gram-positive bacteria, sulconazole has proven to be effective in impetigo and ecthyma.[51]

Fenticonazole

Pharmacology

Fenticonazole is an imidazole derivative with wide spectrum of activity against fungal pathogens. Following topical application, it is poorly absorbed into the systemic circulation. Fenticonazole attains a reservoir effect in the stratum corneum due to prolonged retention time.[52] In common with other azoles, fenticonazole causes indirect inhibition of the ergosterol biosynthesis by inhibiting lanosterol 14α-demethylase. Additionally, it appears to inhibit the release of protease acid by *C. albicans* and blocks cytochrome oxidases and peroxidases.[53]

Spectrum of Activity

Like other azoles, in vitro studies have demonstrated that fenticonazole is active against most dermatophytes, yeasts and molds. Its antifungal activity appears to be affected by pH, with a significant decrease at alkaline pH and in the presence of serum.[54] Additionally, it is also active against gram-positive bacteria such as *S. aureus, S. epidermidis, Streptococcus* species, and *G. vaginalis*, and parasites such as *T. vaginalis*.[55]

Clinical Use

It is available as 2% fenticonazole nitrate cream and solution which have proven to be effective in the treatment of cutaneous fungal infections including dermatophytosis, cutaneous candidiasis and pityriasis versicolor.[56] Fenticonazole is also available as 200 mg and 600 mg vaginal capsules for the treatment of vaginal candidiasis in the dose of 600 mg or 1 g as a single dose or 200 mg/day for 3 days. It has also been used effectively in the management of mixed vulvovaginal infections with *C. albicans, T. vaginalis* and/or *G. vaginalis*.[57]

TRIAZOLES DERIVATIVES

Terconazole

Pharmacology

Terconazole is a triazole antifungal agent which represents first triazole antifungal drug marketed for human use. Its structure is analogous with ketoconazole except for triazole instead of imidazole heterocyclic ring, and isopropyl group instead of acetamide.[58] Following single intravaginal application of a suppository containing 240 mg of terconazole, about 10% is absorbed systemically over a week.

Spectrum of Activity

Terconazole exhibits in vitro antifungal activity against *C. albicans* and *non-albicans Candida* species, dermatophytes, and *C. neoformans*. In vivo studies using animal models have shown terconazole to be effective in the treatment of a variety of dermatomycoses and candidiasis.[58]

Clinical Use

Terconazole, in form of 0.4% and 0.8% vaginal cream and 80 mg vaginal suppositories, are usually indicated for the treatment of vulvovaginal candidiasis. The efficacy of 0.4% terconazole vaginal cream has been shown to be comparable to 0.1% clotrimazole cream in vaginal candidiasis. It is administered as one full applicator (5 g) of 0.4% or 0.8% vaginal cream once daily at bedtime for 7 or 3 consecutive days, respectively. Terconazole 80 mg suppositories are also formulated to be administered intravaginally once daily at bedtime for 3 consecutive days.[59]

Fluconazole

Pharmacology

Fluconazole is a triazole compound with 5-ringed structure containing three nitrogens. The presence of two triazole rings renders it less lipophilic. Further, its antifungal activity is increased by addition of a halogenated phenyl ring. Because of its large molecular weight and hydrophilicity, the bioavailability of intravenous or oral fluconazole is improved but pharmacokinetics become unfavorable for its topical use.[60]

Spectrum of Activity

Topical fluconazole exhibits a broad-spectrum activity against most dermatophytes, *Candida* species, and molds, which is comparable to ketoconazole.[61]

Clinical Use

Fluconazole is commercially available as 0.5% gel form, although newer formulations using microemulsion, nanoemulsion and solid lipid nanoparticles (SLNs) like vehicles have been evaluated to improve the pharmacokinetics of the drug. It has shown good response in the treatment of most superficial cutaneous mycosis such as tinea pedis, tinea cruris, and corporis, cutaneous candidiasis and pityriasis versicolor.[61] Bioadhesive films containing fluconazole have been evaluated for the treatment of mucocutaneous candidiasis.[62]

Efinaconazole

Pharmacology

Efinaconazole is a novel difluorophenyl triazole antifungal agent, available as 10% topical solution (100 mg/g of solution) with good penetration, spreadability and low water solubility. The drug reaches the affected site by transungual as well as subungual route.[63]

Spectrum of Activity

Efinaconazole shows potent activity against most dermatophytic strains, *C. albicans* and *non-albicans Candida* species, *M. furfur*, *A. fumigatus* and *C. neoformans*. Moreover, its activity against *T. mentagrophytes* is unaffected by the presence of serum or keratin unlike most other azoles. Rather, efinaconazole has shown a 7-fold higher free drug concentration in the presence of keratin than both ciclopirox and amorolfine.[64]

Clinical Use

Efinaconazole has been approved for the topical treatment of toenail onychomycosis due to *T. rubrum* and *T. mentagrophytes* as once daily for 48 weeks. Two randomized, double-blind, phase III studies have demonstrated higher efficacy of efinaconazole 10% solution in patients with onychomycosis as compared to placebo.[63]

ADVERSE EFFECTS OF TOPICAL AZOLES

Most of the topical azoles are generally well-tolerated. Less commonly, minor and transient adverse effects have been reported such as local burning, stinging, pruritus, erythema, maceration and urticarial eruptions at the site of application.[31] Allergic contact dermatitis to parent compound or one of the excipients such as propylene glycol or sodium sulfite have been reported less frequently.[65] Rarely, systemic adverse effects such as fever and chills, headache, urticaria and abdominal pain may occur following application of topical azoles. Anaphylaxis and toxic epidermal necrolysis have been reported with terconazole warranting discontinuation of therapy.

CONTRAINDICATIONS

Topical azoles are contraindicated in case of known hypersensitivity to azole compound or any of its excipients.

TOPICAL AZOLES IN PREGNANCY AND LACTATION

In general, topical antifungals can be considered safer in pregnancy than systemic counterparts owing to minimal systemic absorption. Among topical azoles, clotrimazole has been assigned pregnancy category B, while rest of the azoles have been assigned pregnancy category C; animal studies did not show evidence of embryo-fetotoxicity or teratogenicity, whereas human studies are lacking. Clotrimazole and miconazole have shown no embryotoxic potential and can be safely given in pregnancy as twice daily for up to 3 weeks.[66]

Because of the poor systemic absorption, topical azoles are unlikely to adversely affect the nursing infant. However, clinical data regarding the secretion of azoles in human breast milk and their effect on breastfed infants are lacking. Clotrimazole and miconazole may be considered potential alternatives for the management of superficial mycosis in lactation. According to animal studies, efinaconazole was found in milk of nursing rats following repeated subcutaneous administration, therefore, FDA states that efinaconazole should be prescribed to women with caution during lactation.[67]

EMERGING TRENDS IN TOPICAL AZOLES

Newer alternative approaches for topical treatment of cutaneous mycoses are being developed in order to enhance the penetration of the parent drug through the target tissues. Various new carriers such as microemulsion formulations of ketoconazole, clotrimazole, itraconazole and fluconazole have been investigated and proven as successful topical delivery systems in cutaneous fungal infections with good safety profile. Liposome loaded miconazole, SLNs and nanostructured lipid carriers (NLCs) formulations loaded with fluconazole and clotrimazole are few more examples of advanced formulations with a promising role in topical antifungal therapeutics.[68] Commercial 1% gel formulation of itraconazole has also been introduced recently, however, it has yet not been used routinely for the treatment of superficial fungal infections. Moreover, mucoadhesive in situ gel formulations of itraconazole have been prepared and evaluated for vaginal application.[69]

CONCLUSION

Topical azoles are broad-spectrum antifungal agents, widely used for the topical management of superficial cutaneous mycoses. Newer topical azoles with improved pharmacokinetics have proven to be a therapeutic success in the field of antimycotics. Emerging drug delivery systems are being developed to improve the pharmacokinetics of drugs so as to attain better therapeutic response.

REFERENCES

1. Havlickova B, Czaika VA, Friedrich M. Epidemiological trends in skin mycoses worldwide. *Mycoses.* 2008;51 Suppl 4:2-15.
2. Poojary S. Topical antifungals: a review and their role in current management of dermatophytoses. *Clin Dermatol Rev.* 2017;1(3):24-9.
3. Maertens JA. History of the development of azole derivatives. *Clin Microbiol Infect Dis.* 2004;10 (Suppl 1):1-10.
4. Ghannoum MA, Rice LB. Antifungal agents: mode of action, mechanisms of resistance, and correlation of these mechanisms with bacterial resistance. *Clin Microbiol Rev.* 1999;12(4):501-17.
5. Rosen T, Schell BJ, Orengo I. Anti-inflammatory activity of antifungal preparations. *Int J Dermatol.* 1997;36(10):788-92.
6. Elgarhy O. An overview of the azoles of interest. *Int J Curr Pharm Res.* 2015;7:1-6.
7. Khabnadideh S, Rezaei Z, Ghasemi Y, Montazeri-Najafabady N. Antibacterial activity of some new azole compounds. *Anti-Infect Agents.* 2012;10(1):26-33.
8. Fromtling RA. Overview of medically important antifungal azole derivatives. *Clin Microbiol Rev.* 1988;1(2):187-217.
9. Shadomy S. In vitro antifungal activity of clotrimazole (Bay b 5097). *Infect Immun.* 1971;4(2):143-8.
10. Sawyer PR, Brogden RN, Pinder RM, Speight TM, Avery. Clotrimazole: a review of its antifungal activity and therapeutic efficacy. *Drugs.* 1975;9(6):424-47.
11. Tamura S, Kuramoto H, Yamada T, Majima H, Miyamoto H. The therapy of candida vaginitis and candida vulvovaginitis with a new antimycotic substance, clotrimazole. *Curr Med Res Opin.* 1973;1(9):540-6.
12. Owens NJ, Nightingale CH, Schweizer RT, et al. Prophylaxis of oral candidiasis with clotrimazole troches. *Arch Intern Med.* 1984;144(2):290-3.
13. Van Cutsem JM, Thienpont D. Miconazole, a broad-spectrum antimycotic agent with antibacterial activity. *Chemotherapy.* 1972;17(6):392-404.
14. Fischman O, de Camargo ZP. Miconazole nitrate in the treatment of dermatomycoses. *Mykosen.* 1974;17(10):251-5.
15. Thienpont D, Van Cutsem J, Van Gerven F, Heeres J, Janssen PA. Ketoconazole—a new broad spectrum orally active antimycotic. *Experientia.* 1979;35(5):606-7.
16. Daneshmend TK, Warnock DW. Clinical pharmacokinetics of ketoconazole. *Clin Pharmacokinet.* 1988;14(1):13-34.
17. Lester M. Ketoconazole 2 percent cream in the treatment of tinea pedis, tinea cruris, and tinea corporis. *Cutis.* 1995;55(3):181-3.
18. Savin RC, Horwitz SN. Double-blind comparison of 2% ketoconazole cream and placebo in the treatment of tinea versicolor. *J Am Acad Dermatol.* 1986;15(3):500-3.
19. Piérard-Franchimont C, Piérard GE, Arrese JE, De Doncker P. Effect of ketoconazole 1% and 2% shampoos on severe dandruff and seborrhoeic dermatitis: clinical, squamometric and mycological assessments. *Dermatology.* 2001;202(2):171-6.
20. Gerhard I, Ohlhorst D, Eggert-Kruse W, Runnebaum B. Topical one-time therapy with ketoconazole: a double-blind randomized study in vaginal mycosis. *Mycoses.* 1989;32(5):253-65.
21. Heel RC, Brogden RN, Speight TM, Avery GS. Econazole: a review of its antifungal activity and therapeutic efficacy. *Drugs.* 1978;16(3):177-201.
22. Fredriksson T. Treatment of dermatomycoses with topical econazole and clotrimazole. *Curr Ther Res.* 1979;25:590-4.
23. Kates SG, Myung KB, McGinley KJ, Leyden JJ. The antibacterial efficacy of econazole nitrate in interdigital toe web infections. *J Am Acad Dermatol.* 1990;22(4):583-6.
24. Bassiouny A, Kamel T, Moawad MK, Hindawy DS. Broad-spectrum antifungal agents in otomycosis. *J Laryngol Otol.* 1986;100(8):867-73.

25. Croxtall JD, Plosker GL. Sertaconazole: a review of its use in the management of superficial mycoses in dermatology and gynaecology. *Drugs*. 2009;69(3):339-59.

26. Farré M, Ugena B, Badenas JM, et al. Pharmacokinetics and tolerance of sertaconazole in man after repeated percutaneous administration. *Arzneimittelforschung*. 1992;42(5A):752-4.

27. Carrillo-Muñoz AJ, Tur-Tur C, Cárdenes DC, Estivill D, Giusiano G. Sertaconazole nitrate shows fungicidal and fungistatic activities against Trichophyton rubrum, Trichophyton mentagrophytes, and epidermophyton floccosum, causative agents of tinea pedis. *Antimicrob Agents Chemother*. 2011;55(9):4420-1.

28. Liebel F, Lyte P, Garay M, Babad J, Southall MD. Anti-inflammatory and anti-itch activity of sertaconazole nitrate. *Arch Dermatol Res*. 2006;298(4):191-9.

29. Jegasothy BV, Pakes GE. Oxiconazole nitrate: pharmacology, efficacy, and safety of a new imidazole antifungal agent. *Clin Ther*. 1991;13(1):126-41.

30. Polak A. Antifungal activity of four antifungal drugs in the cutaneous retention time test. *Sabouraudia*. 1984;22(6):501-3.

31. Phillips RM, Rosen T. Topical antifungal agents. In: Wolverton SE (Ed). Comprehensive Dermatologic Drug Therapy, 3rd edition. Edinburgh: Saunders Elsevier; 2013. pp. 460-65.

32. Gugnani HC, Ideyi C, Gugnani MK. Oxiconazole in the treatment of tropical dermatomycoses. *Curr Ther Res*. 1993;54(1):122-5.

33. Khanna D, Bharti S. Luliconazole for the treatment of fungal infections: an evidence-based review. *Core Evid*. 2014;9:113-24.

34. Koga H, Nanjoh Y, Makimura K, Tsuboi R. In vitro antifungal activities of luliconazole, a new topical imidazole. *Med Mycol*. 2009;47(6):640-7.

35. Gupta AK, Daigle D. A critical appraisal of once-daily topical luliconazole for the treatment of superficial fungal infections. *Infect Drug Resist*. 2016;9:1-6.

36. Lücker PW, Beubler E, Kukovetz WR, Ritter W. Retention time and concentration in human skin of bifonazole and clotrimazole. *Dermatologica*. 1984;169(Suppl 1):51-5.

37. Lackner TE, Clissold SP. Bifonazole. A review of its antimicrobial activity and therapeutic use in superficial mycoses. *Drugs*. 1989;38(2):204-25.

38. Sanchez JL, Gonzalez J. Clinical management of tinea corporis cruris and tinea pityriasis versicolor two to three week treatment with bifonazole 1%. *Adv Ther*. 1986;3(6):272-80.

39. Marriott MS, Brammer KW, Faccini J, et al. Tioconazole, a new broad-spectrum antifungal agent: preclinical studies related to vaginal candidiasis. *Gynakol Rundsch*. 1983;23(Suppl 1):1-11.

40. Jevons S, Gymer GE, Brammer KW, Cox DA, Leeming MR. Antifungal activity of tioconazole (UK-20,349), a new imidazole derivative. *Antimicrob Agents Chemother*. 1979;15(4):597-602.

41. Clissold SP, Heel RC. Tioconazole. A review of its antimicrobial activity and therapeutic use in superficial mycoses. *Drugs*. 1986;31(1):29-51.

42. Hay RJ, Mackie RM, Clayton YM. Tioconazole nail solution—an open study of its efficacy in onychomycosis. *Clin Exp Dermatol*. 1985;10(2):111-5.

43. Font E, Freixes J, Julve J. Profile of a new topical antimycotic, eberconazole. *Rev Iberoam Micol*. 1995;12(1):16-7.

44. Adimi P, Hashemi SJ, Mahmoudi M, et al. In-vitro activity of 10 antifungal agents against 320 dermatophyte strains using microdilution method in Tehran. *Iran J Pharm Res*. 2013;12(3):537-45.

45. Fernández-Torres B, Inza I, Guarro J. In vitro activities of the new antifungal drug eberconazole and three other topical agents against 200 strains of dermatophytes. *J Clin Microbiol*. 2003;41(11):5209-11.

46. Repiso Montero T, López S, Rodríguez C, et al. Eberconazole 1% cream is an effective and safe alternative for dermatophytosis treatment: multicenter, randomized, double-blind, comparative trial with miconazole 2% cream. *Int J Dermatol*. 2006;45(5):600-4.

47. Sulconazole—a new antifungal for the skin. *Drug Ther Bull*. 1986;24(17):67-8.

48. Franz TJ, Lehman P. Percutaneous absorption of sulconazole nitrate in humans. *J Pharm Sci*. 1988;77(6):489-91.

49. Benfield P, Clissold SP. Sulconazole. A review of its antimicrobial activity and therapeutic use in superficial dermatomycoses. *Drugs.* 1988;35(2):143-53.

50. Iwata K, Yamamoto Y. Studies on the antifungal activities of sulconazole nitrate II. Influences of various factors on the antifungal activity. *Jpn J Med Mycol.* 1984;25(2):147-57.

51. Nolting S, Strauss WB. Treatment of impetigo and ecthyma. A comparison of sulconazole with miconazole. *Int J Dermatol.* 1988;27(10):716-9.

52. Veronese M, Barzaghi D, Bertoncini A, Cornelli U. Fenticonazole: a new antifungal imidazole derivative in vitro and in vivo antimycotic activity. *Mycoses.* 2009;27(4):194-202.

53. Tumietto F, Giacomelli L. Fenticonazole: an effective topical treatment for superficial mycoses as the first-step of antifungal stewardship program. *Eur Rev Med Pharmacol Sci.* 2017;21(11):2749-56.

54. Costa AL. "In vitro" antimycotic activity of fenticonazole (Rec 15/1476). *Mykosen.* 1982;25(1):47-52.

55. Fontana C, Cammarata E, Greco M, Olivieri S. In vitro activity of fenticonazole on Trichomonas vaginalis and Gardnerella vaginalis. *Curr Ther Res Clin Res.* 1990;48:44-51.

56. Sartani A, Cordaro CI, Panconesi E. A multicenter trial with a new imidazole derivative, fenticonazole in superficial fungal skin infections. *Curr Ther Res.* 1988;43(6):1194-203.

57. Bukovsky I, Schneider D, Arieli S, Caspi E. Fenticonazole in the treatment of vaginal trichomoniasis and vaginal mixed infections. *Adv Ther.* 1991;8(4):166-71.

58. Heeres J, Hendrickx R, Van Cutsem J. Antimycotic azoles. 6. Synthesis and antifungal properties of terconazole, a novel triazole ketal. *J Med Chem.* 1983;26(4):611-3.

59. Li T, Zhu Y, Fan S, Liu X, et al. A randomized clinical trial of the efficacy and safety of terconazole vaginal suppository versus oral fluconazole for treating severe vulvovaginal candidiasis. *Med Mycol.* 2015;53(5):455-61.

60. Yim SM, Ko JH, Lee YW, et al. Study to compare the efficacy and safety of fluconazole cream with flutrimazole cream in the treatment of superficial mycosis: a multicentre, randomised, double-blind, phase III trial. *Mycoses.* 2010;53(6):522-9.

61. Aste N, Baldari U, Bellini M, et al. Efficacy and safety of the topical formulation of fluconazole 0.5% (gel containing an emulsion oil/water o/w) in the treatment of dermatomycoses with localized lesions: Results of a multicenter, open, non comparative study. *Giornale Italiano di Dermatologia e Venereologia.* 1999:134(1):61-5.

62. Patel SK, Shah DR, Tiwari S. Bioadhesive films containing fluconazole for mucocutaneous candidiasis. *Indian J Pharm Sci.* 2015;77(1):55-61.

63. Elewski BE, Rich P, Pollak R, et al. Efinaconazole 10% solution in the treatment of toenail onychomycosis: Two phase III multicenter, randomized, double-blind studies. *J Am Acad Dermatol.* 2013;68(4):600-8.

64. Lipner S, Scher R. Efinaconazole in the treatment of onychomycosis. *Infect Drug Resist.* 2015;8:163-72.

65. Brans R, Wosnitza M, Baron JM, Merk HF. Contact sensitization to azole antimycotics. *Hautarzt.* 2009; 60(5):372-5.

66. Prabhu SS, Sankineni P. Managing dermatophytoses in pregnancy, lactation, and children. *Clin Dermatol Rev.* 2017;1(3):34-7.

67. LLC VPNA. (2014). Jublia (efinaconazole) topical solution, 10% (Package Insert). Bridgewater, NJ, USA. [online] Available from http://www.accessdata.fda.gov/drugsatfda_docs/label/2014/203567s000lbl.pdf. [Last Accessed February, 2019].

68. Güngör S, Erdal M, Aksu B. New formulation strategies in topical antifungal therapy. *J Cosmet Dermatol Sci Appl.* 2013;3(1A):56-65.

69. Karavana SY, Rençbe S, Şenyiğit ZA, Baloglu E. A new in-situ gel formulation of itraconazole for vaginal administration. *Pharmacol Pharm.* 2012;3:417-26.

World Clin Dermatol. 2019;5(1):101-10.

Hydroxypyridone Topical Antifungal

Sneha Ghunawat MD DNB

Consultant Dermatologist and Cosmetologist, Meraki Skin Clinic
Gurugram, Haryana, India

ABSTRACT

Hydroxypyridone are a class of antimycotic agent that differ from the rest by their unique mechanism of action. The group includes ciclopirox, rilopirox and piroctone olamine. Because of the excellent tolerability and broad spectrum of antimycotic activity, ciclopirox has been used widely in the past as a topical agent for dermatophytic infections, candidiasis and onychomycosis. The unique mechanism of action makes the drug less prone to develop resistance. The current article aims at highlighting the mechanism of action, safety profile and efficacy in clinical trials of this common antimycotic agent.

INTRODUCTION

Hydroxypyridone are weak acids with broad spectrum of activity. Ciclopirox is the prototype drug of this group; newer ones include rilopirox and octopirox (piroctone olamine). Ciclopirox has a chemical formula 6-cyclohexyl-1-hydroxy-4-methyl-1(1H)-pyridone. It is available in various formulations including cream, lotion, suspension, gel and nail lacquer. The cream and lotion contain ciclopirox olamine 1%, while the gel 0.77% is in the form of free acid. These are equivalent in the dosage strengths. Rilopirox has potential use in the treatment of vaginal candidiasis, seborrheic dermatitis and tinea versicolor. However, no clinical studies are available to confirm these indications. Piroctone olamine has clinical uses in mild-to-moderate cases of seborrheic dermatitis. Ciclopirox being the prototype drug in this group shall be discussed extensively in this article.

Email: sneha.ghunawat@gmail.com

Hydroxypyridones differ from the other antimycotic agents by their unique mechanism of action which involves chelation of heavy metals and interference with membrane permeases and membrane integrity. In addition to this, the broad antimycotic activity of the molecule along with anti-inflammatory and antibacterial activity make this compound unique in its effects. These properties make it a suitable agent to be used in scenarios of secondary infection and inflamed superficial mycosis. It has both fungistatic and fungicidal effect. It also has additional advantage of effective penetration into the skin and nail layers. Ciclopirox has been extensively used to treat tinea infection of the skin, pityriasis versicolor, seborrheic dermatitis and onychomycosis.

MECHANISM OF ACTION

Majority of the antifungal agents act by interfering with the synthesis of ergosterol, which is an important constituent of the fungal cell wall. Earlier studies pointed towards chelation of iron and inhibition of iron-dependent enzymes as the mechanism of action of hyroxypyridones. However, recent data suggests that it acts via chelation of polyvalent ions such as iron and aluminium. This leads to inhibition of metal dependent enzymes such as catalase and cytochromes that are important in cellular activity. Genomic transcriptional assays have shown alteration in levels of iron permeases and proteins involved in iron metabolism.[1] Metabolic activity, oxygen availability and iron levels are critical parameters in the mode of action. Electron microscopic analysis has shown ultrastructural changes such as disorganization of internal structure and cell wall disruption in fungal cell wall of patients with pityriasis versicolor.[2] Another proposed mechanism of action of ciclopirox in mucosal candidal infection is its inhibitory activity of aspartyl proteinases, which has a role in adhesion of yeast cells to the epithelial cells.

Anti-inflammatory and Antiallergic Properties

Ciclopirox is shown to inhibit the arachidonic acid cascade thus exerting an anti-inflammatory and anti-allergic effect. It inhibits prostaglandin and leukotriene synthesis in human polymorphonuclear cells. Inhibition of 5-lipoxygenase and cyclooxygenase also contributes to the anti-inflammatory activity of the drug. Anti-inflammatory effect of the drug has been attributed to decrease in reactive oxygen species by chelating metals such as iron and copper and also scavenging hydroxyl radical.[3,4] The anti-inflammatory activity of ciclopirox has added an advantage in treating fungal infections. The free fatty acids released by the *Malassezia* species lead to free radical generation by the cells. The anti-inflammatory effect of the molecule has added therapeutic effect in condition like seborrheic dermatitis caused by *Malassezia* species.[5] Its anti-inflammatory activity has been shown to be similar to the reference anti-inflammatory agents such as indomethacin and desoximetasone.

This property of the drug gains superiority when treating inflammatory conditions such as cutaneous candidiasis and inflammatory dermatophytic infection. In a randomized double-blind trial comparing the efficacy of 1% ciclopirox olamine cream with 1% clotrimazole cream, 96 patients with cutaneous candidiasis were evaluated. Final cure rates at 2 weeks post-treatment were 76% and 63% in the ciclopirox and clotrimazole group, respectively. Significantly greater number of patients were rated as clinically cured at week 1, 2, 3 than those receiving clotrimazole (p <0.05).[6]

In a double-blind multicentric study evaluating the efficacy of 1% clotrimazole cream versus 1% ciclopirox cream in inflammatory tinea pedis showed better response of the inflammatory component in ciclopirox group. Clinical and mycological cure rates were higher at week 2, 3 and 5, 6 post-treatment in the ciclopirox group (p <0.05).[7]

Antibacterial Activity

Ciclopirox has been shown to possess antibacterial activity against gram-positive, gram-negative bacteria, *Mycoplasma* species and *Trichomonas vaginalis*. Its antibacterial activity is superior as compared to the other antimycotic agents.

Human Immunodeficiency Virus Inhibiting Activity

Ciclopirox has demonstrated inhibitory activity against HIV and sexually transmitted infections (STIs) causing pathogens. It inhibits expression of promoter of HIV 1 and also interferes with the hydroxylation step in the hypusine modification of eukaryotic translation initiation factor 5A.[8]

Antitumor Effect

It has been shown to inhibit cell growth and viability in malignant leukemia, myeloma and solid tumor cells. It arrests cell cycle at G1/S phase boundary. Its effect on inhibition of cell proliferation and angiogenesis is attributed to inhibition of deoxyhypusine hydroxylase.

Antiplasmodial Activity

Ciclopirox has shown inhibitory activity in *Plasmodium falciparum* cell culture. Antimalarial activity of the drug has been attributed to inhibition of deoxyhypusine hydroxylase.[9]

PHARMACOKINETIC PROPERTY

Dermal Penetration

In vitro experiments using porcine model demonstrated complete inhibition of *T. mentagrophytes* in the lower layer of stratum corneum, following 1 hour of exposure to ciclopirox ointment.[9] In a similar study using pig skin model, 100% growth inhibition of *T. mentagrophytes* was noted at the surface following 3 hours of drug exposure. Growth inhibition at stratum granulosum was 93%. None of the azole antimycotics had inhibition above 50% in the deeper layers.[10] Experimental studies using cadaverous human skin showed high concentration of the drug in the dermis 1–2 hour after the application. Concentration of the drug as measured by the radioactivity was found to be highest on the skin surface and hair follicles.[11,12] Concentration gradually decreased with increasing depth, yet levels above the minimum inhibitory concentration were noted in the upper dermis. Drug is absorbed in concentration of 1.3–2.4% in the systemic circulation and is renally excreted as glucuronide.

Intravaginal Administration

Two studies were performed to measure the systemic absorption of ciclopirox following intravaginal application of 2% douche or vaginal pessaries. Systemic absorption in the range of 7–9% was estimated following few hours of absorption.[13]

Nail Application

Penetration of ciclopirox has been studied in the nail following in vivo and in vitro studies with radiolabeled ciclopirox nail lacquer. Concentration achieved in the nail bed exceeded the minimum inhibitory concentration (MIC) for most of the onychomycosis causing dermatophytes. Concentration gradient of 8 μg/mg in the upper layer to 0.03 μg/mg in the deeper layers.[14] Thus effective concentrations of the drug were noted throughout the nail unit.

ANTIFUNGAL SPECTRUM

Ciclopirox demonstrates broad spectrum of activity as an antimycotic agent. It acts as both fungistatic and fungicidal agent depending on the concentration reached in target cells. It is effective against dermatophytes, yeast, actinomycetes, eumycetes and dimorphic fungi (Table 1).[15] It demonstrates fungicidal activity against non-growing fungal cells, which is particularly suitable when treating onychomycosis.

Table 1: Common Fungal Species Against which Ciclopirox has in vitro Susceptibility	
Dermatophytes	• *Trichophyton mentagrophytes*
	• *T. rubrum*
	• *T. verrucosum*
	• *T. tonsurans*
	• *T. soudanense*
	• *T. violaceum*
	• *Microsporum canis*
	• *M. gypseum*
	• *Epidermophyton floccosum*
Yeasts	• *Candida albicans*
	• *C. tropicalis*
	• *C. parapsilosis*
	• *Cryptococcus neoformans*
	• *Malassezia* species
	• *Saccharomyces cerevisiae*
	• *Torulopsis glabrata*
Dimorphic fungi	• *Blastomyces dermatitidis*
	• *Histoplasma capsulatum*
Eumycetes	• *Madurella grisea*
	• *M. mycetomi*
	• *Petriellidium boydii*
Actinomycetes	• *Nocardia asteroides*
	• *N. brasiliensis*
Others	• *Aspergillus* species
	• *Penicillium* species
	• *Phialophora* species
	• *Fusarium solani*

The fungicidal activity against *Trichophyton mentagrophytes* was measured after 1 hour of drug exposure. The antimycotics showed the following efficacy:

Ciclopirox cream 1% > Naftifine cream 1% > Oxiconazole cream 1% > Bifonazole cream 1%.[11]

It also has superior activity against *C. albicans* compared to other antimycotic. Ultrafiltration tissue activity was used to test the antifungal activity of the agents. The relative antifungal activity of the agents tested was as follows:

Tioconazole, oxiconazole, miconazole, econazole, clotrimazole, bifonazole and naftifine creams.[11]

Common available formulations of ciclopirox:

- Shampoo: 1%, 1.5%
- Cream: 1%
- Gel: 0.77%
- Nail lacquer: 8%.

EFFICACY IN CLINICAL TRIALS

Tinea Versicolor

In a study with 90 patients suffering from pityriasis versicolor, ciclopirox olamine 0.1% solution was applied twice daily for 4 weeks. Following 4 weeks of treatment, 74% achieved clinical cure, further 4 weeks of treatment increased the cure rate to 86%.[16] In a double-blind randomized control trial, ciclopirox olamine 1% cream was compared with vehicle for the treatment of pityriasis versicolor. Following 2 weeks of twice daily application of the drug, superior cure rates were achieved with ciclopirox as compared with the vehicle. Total of 49% of patients achieved clinical and mycological cure, compared to 24% in the control group (p <0.0001).[17]

Seborrheic Dermatitis

Multiple topical formulations containing ketoconazole, zinc pyrithione and ciclopirox have been used successfully for the treatment of seborrheic dermatitis for many years. Various trials have pointed toward the advantages of ciclopirox over other topical drugs in terms of persistence of improvement and lower adverse effects. In a randomized open label study comparing the effect of ciclopirox versus ketoconazole in the treatment and long-term effectiveness in seborrheic dermatitis, reported greater response to ciclopirox (p = 0.03) compared to 2% ketoconazole.[18]

In a study comparing the efficacy of piroctone olamine/climbazole shampoo with zinc pyrithione shampoo in patients with mild-to-moderate dandruff, the first group showed higher antimycotics substantively compared to the second. The former group also provided better cosmetic and hair conditioning benefits.[19]

Dermatophytic Infections

In a comparative trial of ciclopirox versus clotrimazole in the treatment of tinea pedis, the drug was applied twice daily for 4 weeks in both the groups. Significantly better clinical cure rates were noted in the ciclopirox group both during the treatment as well as post therapy. At the end of 6 weeks, the combined as well as the mycological cure rates in the ciclopirox group were better than the clotrimazole group (p <0.05).[7]

Vulvovaginal Candidiasis

Vulvovaginal candidiasis, presents with symptoms of vulvar pruritus, dyspareunia, curdy white vaginal discharge and soreness. The most common pathogen implicated in the infection is *Candida albicans* followed by *C. glabrata* and *C. tropicalis*. The recent trend in the infection demonstrates the rising incidence of non-*Candida albicans* candidiasis, as well as resistance of the pathogen against the commonly used antimycotics such as azoles, polyene and echinocandins. Ciclopirox has been used as a successful antimycotic agent for the treatment of VVC.

In addition to the broad spectrum of antifungal activity of ciclopirox against the *Candida* species, it is also effective against the azole resistant species of *Candida* like *C. glabrata*, *C. krusei* due to its unique mode of action. This also makes it a favorable option in conditions of recurrent candidal infection. The inhibitory activity of ciclopirox against *Gardnerella vaginalis* and *Trichomonas vaginalis* makes it a suitable choice when dealing with mixed infection of the female genital tract.

Extravaginal Candidiasis

In a randomized control trial comparing the efficacy of 1% ciclopirox cream versus 1% clotrimazole cream and placebo in the treatment of cutaneous candidiasis, the former demonstrated superior efficacy in the treatment of the infection. The assigned drugs were applied twice daily for 4 weeks. Significantly better clinical cure rated were seen in the ciclopirox treated group compared to clotrimazole group. However, the mycological cure rates were similar in the two groups. This may be attributed to the anti-inflammatory activity of ciclopirox in ameliorating the clinical manifestations of inflammation.[20]

Onychomycosis

Randomized control trial comparing water soluble ciclopirox 8% formulation in hydroxypropyl chitosan to amorolfine 5% lacquer in the treatment of mild-to-moderate onychomycosis, superior results were noted with ciclopirox. The former group showed statistically higher cure rates at 48 weeks and fungal eradication at 24 weeks.[21]

Gupta et al.[22] summarized two pivotal US studies. The combined results showed 34% mycological cure rate and 8% clinical cure rate versus 10% and 1% in the placebo group respectively. The authors also summarized 13 non-US trials yielding a cure rate of 52.6%. The difference in the results can be explained by the difference in the endpoints among the various studies.

ADVERSE EFFECTS

The incidence of adverse effects following topical use of the medication is infrequent (<5% of treated patients). Most common among them are burning sensation, pruritus, pain etc. The burning sensation following the gel application is probably due to the isopropyl alcohol content of the formulation.

The safety of intra vaginal application of ciclopirox has been reviewed in many clinical trials. Adverse effects reported were mild and self-limiting.

The ciclopirox nail lacquer has shown good tolerability. Mild adverse effects reported include periungual redness and tingling sensation.

Many tests have been performed in the animals to detect any carcinogenic, mutagenic and dysmorphogenic effects of the drug. The studies did not report any potential for any of these adverse effects. The drug also did not display any teratogenic or embryotoxic effects.[16]

SAFETY DURING PREGNANCY AND LACTATION

Studies have been performed on animal models at doses 10 times higher than the standard dose used for humans to study the teratogenic potential of the drug. It was not found to have any significant adverse effect. However controlled studies in pregnant women are lacking. It is a pregnancy category B drug and is also considered safe to be used in children more than 10 years of age.[23]

No studies have been conducted so far to study the safety of ciclopirox during breastfeeding. Since only about 1.3% of the drug is absorbed in the blood, it is considered low risk for the nursing infant. Only water miscible creams and gels are to be used by the lactating mother; ointment preparations because of the high level of mineral paraffins are not safe for the licking infants.[24]

CONCLUSION

Hydroxypyridone is class of antifungal with multi-level mechanism of action. They act as metal chelators, decrease level of membrane transporters and increase cellular oxidation. The unique mechanism of action decreases the incidence of resistance. No study till yet have reported resistance with the use of ciclopirox. In its use over the past 20–30 years, it has been found be safe and effective as a broad spectrum antimycotic and antibacterial agent.

REFERENCES

1. Niewerth M, Kunze D, Seibold M, Schaller M, Korting HC, Hube B. Ciclopirox olamine treatment affects the expression pattern of Candida albicans genes encoding virulence factors, iron metabolism proteins, and drug resistance factors. *Antimicrob Agents Chemother.* 2003;47:1805-17.
2. Sigle HC, Thewes S, Niewerth M, Korting HC, Schäfer-Korting M, Hube B. Oxygen accessibility and iron levels are critical factors for the antifungal action of ciclopirox against Candida albicans. *J Antimicrob Chemother.* 2005;55:663-73.
3. Rosen T, Schell BJ, Orengo I. Anti-inflammatory activity of antifungal preparations. *Int J Dermatol.* 1997;36:788-92.
4. Lassus A, Nolting KS, Savopoulos C. Comparison of ciclopirox olamine 1% cream with ciclopirox 1%-hydrocortisone acetate 1% cream in the treatment of inflamed superficial mycoses. *Clin Ther.* 1988;10:594-9.
5. Sato E, Kohno M, Nakashima T, Niwano Y. Ciclopirox olamine directly scavenges hydroxyl radical. *Int J Dermatol.* 2008;47:15-8.
6. Jue SG, Dawson GW, Brogden RN. Ciclopirox olamine 1% cream. A preliminary review of its antimicrobial activity and therapeutic use. *Drugs.* 1985;29:330-41.
7. Evaluation of ciclopirox olamine cream for the treatment of tinea pedis: multicenter, double-blind comparative studies. *Clin Ther.* 1985;7:409-17.
8. Hoque M1, Hanauske-Abel HM, Palumbo P, Saxena D, D'Alliessi Gandolfi D, Park MH, et al. Inhibition of HIV-1 gene expression by Ciclopirox and Deferiprone, drugs that prevent hypusination of eukaryotic initiation factor 5A. *Retrovirology.* 2009;6:90.
9. Saeftel M, Sarite RS, Njuguna T, Holzgrabe U, Ulmer D, Hoerauf A, et al. Piperidones with activity against Plasmodium falciparum. *Parasitol Res.* 2006;99:281-6.
10. Hanel H, Raether W, Dittmar W. Evaluation of fungicidal action in vitro and in a skin model considering the influence of penetration kinetics of various standard antimycotics. *Ann N Y Acad Sci.* 1988;544:329-37.
11. Aly R, Maibach HI, Bagatell FK, Dittmar W, Hänel H, Falanga V, et al. Ciclopirox olamine lotion 1%: bioequivalence to ciclopirox olamine cream 1% and clinical efficacy in tinea pedis. *Clin Ther.* 1989;11:290-303.
12. Kligman AM, McGinley KJ, Foglia A. An in vitro human skin model for assaying topical drugs against dermatophytic fungi. *Acta Derm Venereol.* 1987;67:243-8.
13. Coppi G, Silingardi S, Girardello R, De Aloysio D, Manzardo S. Pharmacokinetics of ciclopirox olamine after vaginal application to rabbits and patients. *J Chemother.* 1993;5:302-6.
14. Monti D. In vitro transungual permeation of ciclopirox from a hydroxypropyl chitosan-based, water-soluble nail lacquer. *Drug Dev Ind Pharm.* 2005;31:11-7.
15. Gupta AK, Skinner AR. Ciclopirox for the treatment of superficial fungal infections: a review. *Int J Dermatol.* 2003;42:3-9.
16. Korting HC, Grundmann-Kollmann M. The hydroxypyridones: a class of antimycotics of its own. *Mycoses.* 1997;40:243-7.
17. Treatment of tinea versicolor with a new antifungal agent, ciclopirox olamine cream 1%. *Clin Ther.* 1985;7:574-83.
18. Chosidow O, Maurette C, Dupuy P. Randomized, open-labeled, non-inferiority study between ciclopiroxolamine 1% cream and ketoconazole 2% foaming gel in mild to moderate facial seborrheic dermatitis. *Dermatology.* 2003;206:233-40.

19. Schmidt-Rose T, Braren S, Fölster H, Hillemann T, Oltrogge B, Philipp P, et al. Efficacy of a piroctone olamine/climbazol shampoo in comparison with a zinc pyrithione shampoo in subjects with moderate to severe dandruff. *Int J Cosmet Sci.* 2011;33:276-82.

20. Evaluation of a new antifungal cream, ciclopirox olamine 1% in the treatment of cutaneous candidosis. *Clin Ther.* 1985;8:41-8.

21. Iorizzo M, Hartmane I, Derveniece A, Mikazans I. Ciclopirox 8% HPCH Nail Lacquer in the Treatment of Mild-to-Moderate Onychomycosis: A Randomized, Double-Blind Amorolfine Controlled Study Using a Blinded Evaluator. *Skin Appendage Disord.* 2016;1:134-40.

22. Gupta AK, Fleckman P, Baran R. Ciclopirox nail lacquer topical solution 8% in the treatment of toenail onychomycosis. *J Am Acad Dermatol.* 2000;43:S70-80.

23. Patel VM, Schwartz RA, Lambert WC. Topical antiviral and antifungal medications in pregnancy: a review of safety profiles. *J Eur Acad Dermatol Venereol.* 2017;31:1440-6.

24. Leachman SA, Reed BR. The use of dermatologic drugs in pregnancy and lactation. *Dermatol Clin.* 2006;24:167-97.

World Clin Dermatol. 2019;5(1):111-26.

Antifungal Resistance: What We Know

[1,]*Surabhi Sinha MD DNB MNAMS, [2]Rashmi Sarkar MD MNAMS

[1]Department of Dermatology and STD, Dr Ram Manohar Lohia Hospital and
Postgraduate Institute of Medical Education and Research, New Delhi, India
[2]Department of Dermatology, STD and Leprosy, Maulana Azad Medical College and
Lok Nayak Hospital, New Delhi, India

ABSTRACT

Antifungal failure has increasingly become a major concern for most dermatologists treating dermatophytoses. Failure to completely respond could be due to various factors either drug-, host-, or environment-related. Antifungal resistance is one of the reasons, though how big a concern it is, remains to be seen. This article focusses on what is currently known on antifungal resistance along with the treatment options in such cases. The current situation needs more scienitifc use of existing drugs and formulations, along with better documentation and identification of the dermatophyte species and its resistance testing for better treatment strategies.

INTRODUCTION

The prevalence of dermatophytoses has been consistently on the rise in the recent few years in India, ranging from 36% to 78%.[1] Different clinical presentations, atypical sites, decreased therapeutic responses and chronicity of the lesions further complicate the scenario. A seemingly innocuous easy-to-treat disease has now become the Achilles' heel for all dermatologists across the country. Surprisingly, this change in prevalence is not mirrored in other neighboring nations like Pakistan, Sri Lanka, Nepal or even Turkey and Iran.

Before we delve deeper into the reasons for this phenomenon, we need to apprise ourselves of certain relevant terminologies.[2,3]

*Corresponding author
Email: surabhi2310@gmail.com

- *Naïve dermatophytosis*—defined as one in which the subject has never been previously exposed to a particular infection or to treatment for that infection
- *Chronic dermatophytosis*—the subject has suffered from the disease more than 6 months with/without recurrence, in spite of adequate treatment
- *Recurrent dermatophytosis*—recurrence of lesions within 4–6 weeks of completion of treatment with at least two such episodes in last 6 months
- *Relapse of dermatophytosis*—recurrence of lesions after 6–8 weeks of completion of treatment (implying the infection has been acquired from an unnoticed site like nail, vellus hair, etc.).

Approximately 5–10% to 15–20% of cases are recurrent or chronic cases.[3,4]

The point-of-care testing (POCT) recommended by the Expert consensus group on dermatophytosis (ECTODERM India) for confirmation of the diagnosis is 10% potassium hydroxide (KOH) mount of the skin scraping and observing it 15–30 minutes after preparation for higher sensitivity.[2] They also recommended dermoscopy (to look for vellus hair involvement as an indicator both of possible relapse and of systemic therapy) and fungal culture in recalcitrant and multisite tinea cases.

CHANGE IN PRESENTATION

The most common presentations are tinea cruris and tinea corporis. Others include tinea capitis, tinea pedis and onychomycosis. The most common species are *Trichophyton rubrum*, *Trichophyton mentagrophytes* and *Microsporum canis*. These are also the species responsible for most cases with atypical presentations too. Atypical presentations of dermatophytoses seen increasingly include:

- Widespread extensive disease
- Atypical morphology—seborrheic dermatitis like psoriasiform, eczematous, lupus like purpuric, pustular, follicular, deep dermal nodules and ulcers in immunocompromised, tinea pseudoimbricata, rosacea-like, etc.
- Atypical age—morphology combinations
- Atypical sites—scalp in adults, face in children and infants, combination of tinea cruris and tinea corporis, extension to scalp and face from truncal lesions
- Decreased response to commonly used drugs (treatment failure)
- Recurrences/relapses/chronic infections.

Steroid-modified tinea (Figures 1 and 2) deserves a special mention at this point, owing to the sheer numbers that abound in dermatology outpatient departments. This could be due to the fact that despite constant objection by the dermatology fraternity, steroid topical preparations continue to be an over-the-counter (OTC) product, easily available and readily prescribed by the "friendly

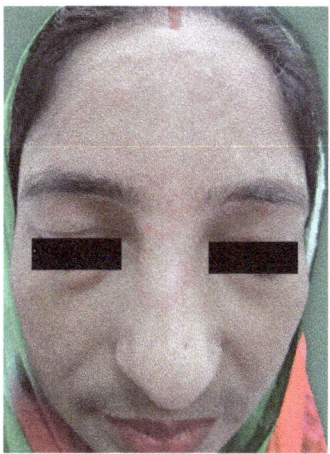

Figure 1: Steroid-modified tinea face.

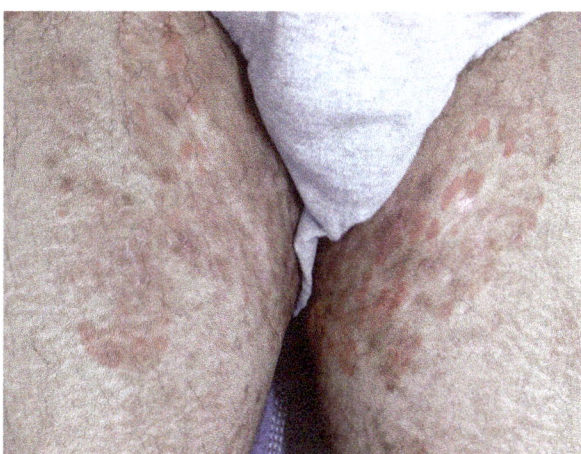

Figure 2: Steroid damage with tinea. *Courtesy:* Dr Konchok Dorjay, Senior Resident, PGIMER and Dr RML Hospital, New Delhi, India.

neighborhood" chemists. Some potent topical steroids are also under price control in India, leading to greater potential for misuse and overuse. Steroid use can lead to significant changes in morphology of dermatophytoses:

- Decreased scaling of the lesions
- No active raised margins of the lesions
- Relapse soon after treatment is stopped
- Marked purulent folliculitis.

REASONS FOR CHANGING EPIDEMIOLOGY OF DERMATOPHYTOSES

These are the subject of many a study nowadays, but despite a multitude of factors being held responsible, this is still a gray area. The factors include pathogen, host and environmental factors.

Pathogen Factors

- *Species shift*: Anthropophilic species that colonize humans (e.g. *T. rubrum, T. interdigitale, T. tonsurans*) tend to be associated with more chronic and less inflammatory infections. On the other hand, zoophilic species of dermatophytes (*T. mentagrophytes var. mentagrophytes, T. verrucosum*) often cause highly inflamed lesions. It is possible that a species shift from the prevailing *T. rubrum* to *T. mentagrophytes/T. interdigitale* could be responsible for a change in susceptibility of the fungus to known antifungals. This is postulated to be a cause as a few recent mycological studies undertaken across the country have demonstrated *T. mentagrophytes* or *T. interdigitale* as the predominant organism (Table 1). *Trichophyton mentagrophytes* versus *T. interdigitale*—the debate continues.

  There is confusion prevailing over the nomenclature of the species isolated and designated as "*T. mentagrophytes*" by some laboratories—it is a zoonotic organism and chronic/recalcitrant infections are unlikely to be caused by it. It is more likely to cause widespread, acutely inflammatory pustular, short-lived infections.

  Trichophyton interdigitale was previously classified under the species "*T. mentagrophytes*" as *T. mentagrophytes var. interdigitale* and is more likely to be the cause, being an anthropophilic organism like *T. rubrum*.

  When culture morphology is used for identification—only *T. mentagrophytes complex* can be concluded. For identification of *T. interdigitale*, "you have to look for it if you want to find it". Urease test can be performed; there is difference in the appearance of colonies on 1% Peptone agar and in the pigment pattern on Littman Oxgall Agar too. Microscopic morphology too can be differentiated by the eye of a discerning microbiologist. However, the differentiation is based on a single-base pair difference in the internal transcribed spacer (ITS) region—which is the most widely sequenced deoxyribonucleic acid (DNA) region in molecular ecology of fungi and has been recommended as the universal fungal barcode sequence[14]

- *Antifungal resistance*: Most existing studies do not show much interspecies difference in susceptibility to individual drugs. But more studies are needed with correct strain typing and use of standardized nomenclature. With the

Table 1: List of Predominant Dermatophyte Species Isolated in Studies Published in India in the Last 4 Years

Authors	Year	Part of India	Species
Lakshmanan	2015	South	*T. rubrum > T. mentagrophytes*
Penmetcha et al.	2016	South	*T. rubrum > T. mentagrophytes*
Ramaraj et al.	2016	South	*T. rubrum > T. mentagrophytes*
Poluri et al.	2015	South	*T. rubrum > T. mentagrophytes*
Ganeshkumar et al.	2015	South	*T. rubrum > T. mentagrophytes*
Sudha et al.	2016	South	*T. rubrum > T. mentagrophytes*
Noronha et al.[5]	2016	South	*T. mentagrophytes*
Parmeshwari et al.	2015	South	*T. rubrum > T. mentagrophytes*
Venkatesh et al.[6]	2016	South	*T. mentagrophytes > T. rubrum*
Manjunath et al.	2016	South	*T. rubrum > T. mentagrophytes*
Janardhan et al.	2017	South	*T. rubrum > T. mentagrophytes*
Aruna et al.	2017	South	*T. rubrum > T. mentagrophytes*
Putta et al.[7]	2016	West	*T. mentagrophytes*
Naglot et al.	2015	Northeast	*T. rubrum > T. mentagrophytes*
Sharma et al.[8]	2017	Northeast	*T. mentagrophytes*
Verma et al.[9]	2017	North	*T. mentagrophytes*
Bhatia et al.[10]	2014	North	*T. mentagrophytes > T. rubrum*
Kucheria et al.	2015	North	*T. rubrum > T. mentagrophytes*
Gupta et al.	2014	Central	*T. rubrum*
Majid et al.	2016	North	*T. rubrum > T. tonsurans > T. mentagrophytes*
Khurana et al.[11]	2018	North	*T. interdigitale*
Singh et al.[12]	2018	North	*T. interdigitale > T. rubrum (sequencing of ITS used)*
Mishra et al.[13]	2018	North	*T. mentagrophytes > T. rubrum > T. violaceum*

current confusing nomenclature, any interpretation of laboratory-based data is to be done extremely cautiously
- Dormant fungi
- Role of biofilms—under evaluation—may allow persistence of infection
- Role of mannans—under evaluation
- Role of melanin—being researched
- A vicious cycle comes into play as depicted in Figure 3[15]
- Virulence factors may have changed with/without species shift (Table 2).

The following four steps are involved in the pathogenesis of dermatophytosis:
1. Adherence
2. Germination and growth

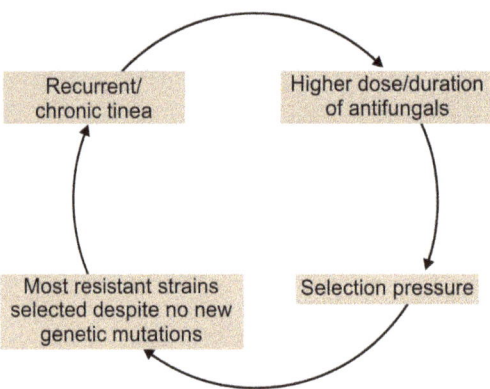

Figure 3: A vicious cycle.

Table 2: Dermatophyte Virulence Factors[16]	
Enzymatic	**Nonenzymatic**
• Protease	• Hemolysis
• Lipase	• Complete hemolysis by all three *Trichophyton* species
• Keratinase	• Hemolysins degrade macrophages and neutrophils
• Phospholipase	
• Gelatinase	• Xanthomegnin
• Elastase	• Melanin—bind to antifungal agents

3. Penetration
4. *Local immune response*: T helper 1 (Th1) and T helper 17 (Th17)-mediated CMI elimination of dermatophyte occurs. Th1 responses confer protection while Th2 responses are nonprotective/associated with disease progression. A triad of chronic dermatophytosis, atopy and immediate hypersensitivity (IH) to *Trichophyton* suggests involvement of Th2 cells. Neutrophil and macrophage are the main effector cells. The first three steps (adherence, germination and penetration) are almost similar in all dermatophytes. The local immune response may change with change in the species (Figure 4).[17]

Local immune evasion may be achieved by:
• Th1 → Th2 shift
• Immunoglobulin E (IgE), IgG4—increased (like atopic dermatitis)
• Decreased proinflammatory cytokines interleukin (IL)-1β, IL-6, IL-8 (potent neutrophil chemotactic factor), tumor necrosis factor-α (TNF-α), interferon-gamma (IFN-γ), IL-17 (decreased human-β defensin)
• Increased anti-inflammatory cytokines—IL-4, IL-10 (→ Th2 shift)

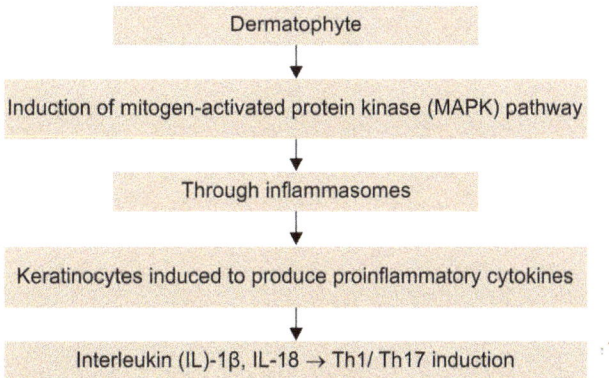

Figure 4: Mechanism of killing of dermatophytes by Th1/Th17-mediated pathway.

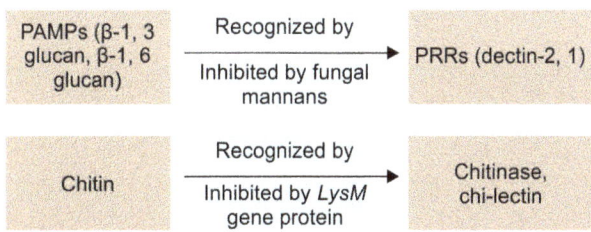

Figure 5: Evasion of pathogen-associated molecular pattern (PAMP)-pattern recognition receptor (PRR) interaction.

- Free radical and NO secretion—low in chronic infections → defective killing
- Downregulation of toll-like receptor 4 (TLR-4) by *T. rubrum* → decreased recruitment of effector cells
- Masking of recognizable fungal cell wall components
- Mannans:
  - Inhibit antigen processing and presentation → defective phagocytosis
  - Block interaction between dendritic cell (DC) and T cells
  - Inhibit dectin-2 recognition of glucans on fungal cell wall
  - Increase IL-10 → anti-inflammatory
  - Decrease rate of Keratinocyte proliferation.
- Glycopeptides:
  - Decreased T lymphocyte proliferation
  - Antigenic interference
  - Evasion of pathogen-associated molecular pattern (PAMP)-pattern recognition receptor (PRR) interaction → becoming "invisible" (Figure 5).

- Role of biofilms—sessile microbial communities surrounded by extracellular polymeric substances (EPS) with increased resistance. *T. rubrum* > *T. menta-grophytes*—more biomass, denser.[18]
  - Too big to be phagocytosed
  - 1%—persisters
  - 10–1,000X increase in minimum inhibitory concentration (MIC)
  - Mechanism of acquired resistance
  - Role in tinea corporis—unknown.

Host Factors

- Change in immune status:
  - Obesity
  - Diabetes mellitus
  - Atopy
  - Immunosuppression
  - Immunodeficiency (CARD9 mutation)
  - Th1/Th2 shift
  - Skin barrier dysfunction.
- Clothing and articles of personal use:
  - Tight clothing
  - Noncotton clothing—occlusion of the skin with nonporous materials interferes skin's barrier function; increase local temperature and hydration
  - Sharing of manicure/pedicure instruments, hats/caps, towels
  - Washing clothes together
  - Sharing bed linen, towels, etc.
- Topical steroid abuse/irrational triple combination prescriptions—one of the most important factors. Topical corticosteroids—help the fungi establish infections by decreasing local CMI (Th1 → Th2, decreased APC of LCs)
- Area of body involved—especially nail/sole involvement, vellus hair involvement
- Broad-spectrum antibiotics
- Noncompliance with treatment
- Cost factor of antifungals
- Tinea of vellus hair more frequent with zoophilic species
- Reinfection from family/fomites ("the new scabies"—ask all family members, treat all symptomatic family members)
- Ignoring pharmacokinetics (PK) and pharmacodynamics (PD) of antifungals—wrong formulation of right antifungal (Itraconazole powder, Amphotericin gel)

- Fomites—*T. mentagrophytes* more than 25 weeks versus *T. rubrum* less than 12 weeks.

Environmental Factors

- Climate change—more warm and humid (does not explain why the change has occurred in India predominantly)
- International travel and migration have increased
- Contact with pets (transmission of animal dermatophytes to humans)
- Untreated/undocumented/undiagnosed family members
- Low socioeconomic status/overcrowding
- Increased use of antifungals in agriculture industry leading to decreased susceptibility.

To further complicate the already bleak situation, there is a severe dearth of data from Indian population due to lack of routine data entry or registries. Additional causes of treatment failure in onychomycosis:

- Drug not reaching the intended site (due to wrong formulation)
- Dermatophytoma refers to a ball of hyperkeratotic mass or clump of dermatophyte hyphae which makes antifungal penetration of antifungal difficult and needs to be removed surgically
- Different species have different susceptibilities
- Dormant arthrospores are more resistant to treatment and provide a reservoir of infection.

TYPES OF FUNGAL RESISTANCE

Resistance can be clinical or microbiological.

- *Clinical resistance* is the failure to eliminate a fungal infection despite the administration of an antifungal agent which may or may not demonstrate MICs in the resistance range for that organism
- *Microbiological resistance* refers to nonsusceptibility of a fungus to an antifungal agent by in vitro susceptibility testing, in which the MIC of the drug exceeds the susceptibility breakpoint for that organism. Microbiological resistance can be primary (intrinsic), where the fungi are resistant to a drug before exposure and secondary (acquired), which develops in response to exposure to an antimicrobial agent. Certain fungal species are intrinsically resistant such as *Candida krusei* to fluconazole and *Cryptococcus neoformans* to echinocandins and nonalbicans *Candida* to 5-flucytosine (5FC). Secondary resistance develops among previously susceptible strains after exposure to the antifungal

agent and is usually dependent on altered gene expression, e.g., terbinafine resistance in *T. rubrum*, fluconazole resistance among *Candida albicans*.

Resistance to antifungals is tested for by in vitro susceptibility testing—most commonly the broth microdilution (BMD) method. The Clinical and Laboratory Standards Institute (CLSI) and the European Committee on Antimicrobial Susceptibility Testing (EUCAST) have laid down certain cutoffs for standardization.

However, MICs have limitations of being tested in vitro and thus being less clinically relevant. Use of *clinical breakpoints* instead of the numerical values of MIC is preferred. Breakpoints are interpretive criteria that are used to denote susceptibility and resistance to antifungal agents.

They are categorized as susceptible, intermediate and resistant—susceptible (the drug is an appropriate treatment); resistant (the drug is not recommended as a treatment), and intermediate/susceptible-dose-dependent (SDD) (the drug may be an appropriate treatment, depending on certain conditions). Basically, clinical breakpoints are the MIC at which a strain behaves as a resistant strain. They are specific for each fungus-drug pair and clinically more significant than MICs.

To determine breakpoints, in vitro microbiological data, PK/PD data of the drug, and outcome data from prospective clinical studies (clinical response vs. MIC value) are needed. The best PK/PD parameter for that species drug pair is taken into consideration. However, in dermatophytes, there is paucity of data in all the three aspects. It is essential to know the prevailing susceptibility and resistance trends to be able to form treatment protocols. Unfortunately, till now, the breakpoints have not been defined for the dermatophytes due to lack of data on the clinical correlation, PK/PD studies, or epidemiological cutoff MIC values.

The "90-60 Rule"

The "90-60 rule" says that susceptible strains respond to antifungals 90% of the times and resistant strains too respond 60% of the times. Thus, resistance, if any, can be combated by increasing the dose further.

RESISTANCE TO SPECIFIC CLASSES OF DRUGS

Naturally occurring resistant mutants in *T. rubrum are believed to be* 10^{-7} for itraconazole and 10^{-9} for terbinafine. Acquired resistance occurs with a 100-fold higher frequency. Itraconazole-resistant mutants cross resistant with other anti-fungals (drug efflux mechanisms); terbinafine-resistant isolates cross resistant only with squalene epoxidase inhibitors and not azoles (target-specific).[19]

Azoles

Azole resistance among dermatophytes has been reported to be as high as 19%. Fluconazole has been reported to have high MICs while eberconazole, luliconazole and itraconazole have low MICs. Innate resistance to ketoconazole and itraconazole was seen in 10% and 15% of patients. Development of acquired resistance and cross resistance among fluconazole and itraconazole was seen after prolonged exposure to low concentrations of these drugs; may cause therapy failures. Mechanism: drug efflux (TruMDR1 and 2), stress adaptation, overexpression of target enzyme.[20-22]

Minimum inhibitory concentration values for itraconazole were significantly lower than fluconazole: high propensity of *T. rubrum* to develop resistance toward fluconazole resulting in treatment failures with this drug. Treatment failure with itraconazole has been noted despite low MICs suggesting role of host factors and drug-related factors. Change of itraconazole from the generic to innovator itraconazole produces improvement in nonresponders. MIC values for itraconazole have been found to be consistently low in most Indian studies and most cases of treatment failure are due to low drug bioavailability.[23]

Allylamines

Traditionally, allylamines have been believed to be superior to azoles for the reasons mentioned here:

- Once a day application
- Rapid onset of action
- Shorter duration of treatment
- Cost-effective
- *Reservoir effect*—sustained cutaneous fungicidal concentration and residual therapeutic activity up to 2–4 weeks post-treatment. Reservoir effect also enables once-daily application
- Traditional azoles are fungistatic and need twice-daily application (not applicable to newer azoles—e.g. eberconazole, luliconazole, sertaconazole)
- Minimal inhibitory concentration of allylamines is equal to, or near their minimal fungicidal concentration, indicating primarily fungicidal activity
- Superior cure rates (both mycological and clinical). Terbinafine has been shown to achieve mycological cure more rapidly than clotrimazole
- Provide residual protection which reduces the relapse rate.

However, MICs to terbinafine have increased recently. Clayton et al. reported MIC of 0.0015–0.01 µg/mL in 1989. However, more recently, Majid et al. reported that 2-week terbinafine therapy led to clinical and microbiological improvement in 65% patients of which 22% relapsed in the 12-week follow-up.[24] Only 43% patients could achieve a long-term clinical and mycological cure. Similarly, Singh et al. reported a 2% cure rate after 2 weeks and 30.6% cure rate after 4 weeks of oral and topical terbinafine.[12] Similar observations have been made from other institutes in northern India.

However, Khurana et al. in their study, found that a higher terbinafine exposure (increased durations/dose) improved outcomes even in those infected with isolates exhibiting MIC greater than or equal to 1 µg/mL.[11] (Cure achieved with standard/higher drug exposure in isolates exhibiting TRB MIC <1 µg/mL: 83.3% and cure achieved with standard/higher drug exposure in isolates exhibiting TRB MIC ≥1 µg/mL: 66.7%.)

Mutations in the target enzyme SQLE were seen in a series of 20 patients, all bearing single nucleotide substitutions in the *SQLE* gene, from 30 isolates with MICs between 4 and 32 µg/mL. The same set of mutations has also been described from another institute in 6 isolates from a total of 20 which were tested. In a correlation study on MICs and SQLE mutations with clinical response to terbinafine: 8 of the 9 patients with less than 50% response to terbinafine in 3 weeks harbored isolates exhibiting elevated TRB MICs (8–32 µg/mL) and SQLE mutations.[25]

Rotta et al. compared two allylamines—naftifine and terbinafine with six azoles—bifonazole, clotrimazole, econazole, fenticonazole, miconazole and oxiconazole. In mycological cure at the end of treatment, 15 trials showed a small difference in favor of allylamines [0.78, 95% confidence interval (CI) 0.48–1.24]. Sustained cure showed a significant result in favor of allylamines (0.55, 95% CI 0.33–0.89).[26]

A meta-analysis involving 14 treatments pooled data of 65 trials. It found that regarding sustained cure outcome, butenafine and terbinafine were significantly more efficacious than clotrimazole, oxiconazole and sertaconazole. Terbinafine also demonstrated statistical superiority when compared with ciclopirox and naftifine showed better response compared with oxiconazole.[27]

Primary terbinafine resistance in T. rubrum: Mukherjee et al. in 2003 due to a single amino acid substitution in SQLE protein (Leu393Phe).

Molecular mechanism of acquired resistance to terbinafine: Point mutations in the *ERG1* gene causing single amino acid substitutions (Leu393, Phe397, Phe415, His440) of the SQLE protein resulting in 100-fold reduced affinity for terbinafine.[28]

Others

- *Ciclopirox and amorolfine* are old drugs but may have a new indication in patients who have already used azoles and allylamines and not responded. Ciclopirox is especially useful in inflammatory tinea and tinea pedis with secondary bacterial infection. An in vitro study of 17 antifungal drugs (terbinafine, naftifine, butenafine, voriconazole, itraconazole, fluconazole, miconazole, amorolfine, tolciclate, clotrimazole, econazole, ketoconazole, ciclopirox olamine, tolnaftate, griseofulvin, undecylenic acid, tioconazole) against a panel of 20 dermatophytes has shown amorolfine as the most active topical agent.[29] However, more randomized controlled trials with long-term follow-up are needed to further study their efficacy in topical treatment of dermatophytosis.

HOW TO MANAGE SUSPECTED RESISTANT DERMATOPHYTOSIS?

General Measures—Tips

- Personal hygiene—most important—bathe twice daily and wipe dry
- Clothing
- Never wear damp clothes
- Wash clothes in hot water (60°C) and dry inside out in the sun/indoors if no sunlight and iron them
- Wash infected clothes separately
- Avoid wearing wrist bands/waist bands
- Wear loose cotton clothes
- Avoid tight synthetic clothes
- Avoid tights/slacks/leggings/jeggings/skinny fit denim clothes
- Regularly wash bed linen
- Avoid sharing bed linen
- Regularly wash caps and socks
- Wear open footwear
- Surrounding environment
- Regular wet mopping followed by floor disinfectant to decrease spores
- Treat all family members who are affected.

TREATMENT PROTOCOLS

- Naïve case:
  - Itraconazole 100 mg twice daily × 4 weeks
  - Terbinafine 250 mg OD × 4–6 weeks
  - Fluconazole 150–200 mg twice weekly × 6–8 weeks.
- Steroid modified:
  - Abrupt stoppage of the steroid being applied should be advised. Itraconazole 200–400 mg daily for 4–6 weeks or longer should be preferred
  - Longer duration of same schedule.

- Recurrences/relapse in 6 months:
  - Give an antifungal that has not been given in the past → for 3 weeks →
    - No response/new lesions → change drug
    - Less response → increase dose.
  - Experts also recommend griseofulvin (250–500 mg twice daily) and fluconazole (150–300 mg/week) in patients who have failed terbinafine or itraconazole. However, delayed clinical response requiring longer duration of treatment should be considered before starting therapy with different drugs.
- Chronic case—longer course up to 3–6 months/up to cure:
  - Combination of oral and topical (e.g. amorolfine and itraconazole seen to be synergistic)
  - It is also advisable to do baseline liver function tests (LFTs) to rule out impaired liver function and periodic follow-up, it treatment duration exceeds 4 weeks.
- Rule of Two:
  - The expert consensus group also endorsed the Rule of Two—"apply topical treatment 2 cm beyond for 2 weeks beyond clinical resolution".[2]
- Systemic therapy should be preferred in case of vellus hair involvement on dermoscopy
- Adjuvant therapies like antihistamines, salicylic acid ad moisturizers play an important role[2]
- In pregnancy, topical antifungals should be the agents of choice in any trimester.[2]

WHAT IS NEW?

The ME1111 is a novel antidermatophytic drug with strong fungicidal properties in nonclinical studies.[30] It is a selective inhibitor of succinate dehydrogenase, a critical enzyme in mitochondrial respiratory electron transfer of *Trichophyton* species. Efficacy has been demonstrated against dermatophytes for which terbinafine or itraconazole MICs are elevated. Treatment of *T. mentagrophytes* dermatophytosis in a guinea pig model showed significantly better clinical efficacy of 10% ME1111 solution than ciclopirox 8% and comparable mycological efficacy.

CONCLUSION

In view of emerging recalcitrance of dermatophytoses, there is an urgent need for better strain typing methods and use of correct standardized universal nomenclature of dermatophytes. Also search for newer/improved/hitherto overlooked virulence factors and use of clinically relevant clinical breakpoints instead of MIC values in antifungal susceptibility testing (AFST) studies should be employed for improved clinical relevance.

REFERENCES

1. Naglot A, Shrimali DD, Nath BK, et al. Recent trends of dermatophytosis in Northeast India (Assam) and interpretation with published studies. *Int J Curr Microbiol App Sci.* 2015;4:111-20.
2. Rajagopalan M, Inamadar A, Mittal A, et al. Expert consensus on the management of dermatophytosis in India (ECTODERM India). *BMC Dermatol.* 2018;18:6.
3. Dogra S, Uprety S. The menace of chronic and recurrent dermatophytosis in India: is the problem deeper than we perceive? *Indian Dermatol Online J.* 2016;7:73-6.
4. Dogra S, Narang T. Emerging atypical and unusual presentations of dermatophytosis in India. *Clin Dermatol Rev.* 2017;1, Suppl S1:12-8.
5. Noronha TM, Tophakhane RS, Nadiger S. Clinico-microbiological study of dermatophytosis in a tertiary-care hospital in North Karnataka. *Indian Dermatol Online J.* 2016;7(4):264-71.
6. Venkatesh VN, Kotian S. Dermatophytosis: a clinico-mycological profile from a tertiary care hospital. *J Int Med Dentist.* 2016;3(2):96-102.
7. Putta SD, Kulkarni VA, Bhadade AA, Kulkarni VN, Walawalkar AS. Prevalence of dermatophytosis and its spectrum in a tertiary care hospital, Kolhapur. *Indian J Basic Appl Med Res.* 2016;5:595-600.
8. Sharma R, Adhikari L, Sharma RL. Recurrent dermatophytosis: a rising problem in Sikkim, a Himalayan state of India. *Indian J Pathol Microbiol.* 2017;60:541-5.
9. Verma S, Verma G, Sharma V, et al. Current spectrum of dermatophytosis in a tertiary care hospital of North India—a 6-year clinico-mycological study. *J Med Sci Clin Res.* 2017;5(3): 19488-94.
10. Bhatia VK, Sharma PC. Epidemiological studies on dermatophytosis in human patients in Himachal Pradesh, India. *Springerplus.* 2014;3:134.
11. Khurana A, Masih A, Chowdhary A, et al. Correlation of in vitro susceptibility based on MICs and squalene epoxidase mutations with clinical response to terbinafine in patients with tinea corporis/cruris. *Antimicrob Agents Chemother.* 2018;62(12). pii: e01038-18.
12. Singh A, Masih A, Khurana A, et al. High terbinafine resistance in Trichophyton interdigitale isolates in Delhi, India harbouring mutations in the squalene epoxidase gene. *Mycoses.* 2018;61(7):477-84.
13. Mishra N, Rastogi MK, Gahalaut P, et al. Clinicomycological study of dermatophytoses in children: presenting at a tertiary care center. *Indian J Paediatr Dermatol.* 2018;19:326-30.
14. Schoch CL, Seifert KA, Huhndorf S, et al. Nuclear ribosomal internal transcribed spacer (ITS) region as a universal DNA barcode marker for fungi. *Proc Natl Acad Sci U S A.* 2012;109(16):6241-6.
15. Hryncewicz-Gwóźdź A, Kalinowska K, Plomer-Niezgoda E, Bielecki J, Jagielski T. Increase in resistance to fluconazole and itraconazole in Trichophyton rubrum clinical isolates by sequential passages in vitro under drug pressure. *Mycopathologica.* 2013;176:49-55.
16. Elavarashi E, Kindo AJ, Rangarajan S. Enzymatic and non-enzymatic virulence activities of dermatophytes on solid media. *J Clin Diagn Res.* 2017;11(2):DC23-5.
17. Woodfolk JA. Allergy and dermatophytes. *Clin Microbiol Rev.* 2005;18(1):30-43.
18. Costa-Orlandi CB, Sardi JC, Santos CT, Fusco-Almeida AM, Mendes-Giannini MJ. In vitro characterization of Trichophyton rubrum and T. mentagrophytes *biofilms*. Biofouling. 2014;30(6):719-27.
19. Ghelardi E, Celandroni F, Gueye SA, et al. Potential of ergosterol synthesis inhibitors to cause resistance or cross-resistance in Trichophyton rubrum. *Antimicrob Agents Chemother.* 2014;58:2825-9.
20. Goh CL, Tay YK, Ali KB, Koh MT, Seow CS. In vitro evaluation of griseofulvin, ketoconazole, and itraconazole against various dermatophytes in Singapore. *Int J Dermatol.* 1994;33: 733-7
21. Hryncewicz-Gwóźdź A, Kalinowska K, Plomer-Niezgoda E, Bielecki J, Jagielski T. Increase in resistance to fluconazole and itraconazole in Trichophyton rubrum clinical isolates by sequential passages in vitro under drug pressure. *Mycopathologia.* 2013;176:49-55.

22. Cervelatti EP, Fachin A, Ferreira-Nozawa M, Martinez-Rossi N. Molecular cloning and characterization of a novel ABC transporter gene in the human pathogen Trichophyton rubrum. *Med Mycol.* 2006;44:141-7.

23. Pierard-Franchimont G, De Doncker P, Van de Velde V, et al. Paradoxical response to itraconazole treatment in a patient with onychomycosis caused by Microsporum gypseum. *Ann Soc Belg Med Trop.* 1995;75:211-7

24. Majid I, Sheikh G, Kanth F, Hakak R. Relapse after oral terbinafine therapy in dermatophytosis: a clinical and mycological study. *Indian J Dermatol.* 2016;61:529-33.

25. Mahajan S, Tilak R, Kaushal SK, Mishra RN, Pandey SS. Clinico-mycological study of dermatophytic infections and their sensitivity to antifungal drugs in a tertiary care center. *Indian J Dermatol Venereol Leprol.* 2017;83:436-40.

26. Rotta I, Sanchez A, Gonçalves PR, Otuki MF, Correr CJ. Efficacy and safety of topical antifungals in the treatment of dermatomycosis: a systematic review. *Br J Dermatol.* 2012;166:927-33.

27. Rotta I, Ziegelmann PK, Otuki MF, et al. Efficacy of topical antifungals in the treatment of dermatophytosis: a mixed-treatment comparison meta-analysis involving 14 treatments. *JAMA Dermatol.* 2013;149:341-9.

28. Yamada T, Maeda M, Alshahni MM, et al. Terbinafine resistance of Trichophyton clinical isolates caused by specific point mutations in the squalene epoxidase gene. Antimicrob *Agents Chemother.* 2017;61:e00115-7.

29. Favre B, Hofbauer B, Hildering KS, Ryder NS. Comparison of in vitro activities of 17 antifungal drugs against a panel of 20 dermatophytes by using a microdilution assay. *J Clin Microbiol.* 2003;41:4817-9.

30. Long L, Hager C, Ghannoum M. Evaluation of the efficacy of ME1111 in the topical treatment of dermatophytosis in a guinea pig model. *Antimicrob Agents Chemother.* 2016;60:2343-5.

World Clin Dermatol. 2019;5(1):127-34.

Newer Topical Antifungals: What Lies Ahead?

Isha Narang MD MRCP (SCE)

Department of Dermatology,
University Hospitals of Derby and Burton, United Kingdom

ABSTRACT

Dermatophytosis has become a blazing epidemic in the recent past. In this scenario, though oral antifungals are the mainstay of therapy, the role of topical antifungals is also crucial. Several new topical antifungal agents and newer formulations have proven to be highly efficacious in the management of fungal infections. We are constantly exploring newer drug characteristics to fight antifungal resistance. The article describes salient features of the commonly used drugs such as efinaconazole, eberconazole, tavobarole along with an update on newer drugs that are under development.

INTRODUCTION

Antifungal resistance is a major issue due to variety of host, agent and environmental factors. We constantly need newer antifungals to break this resistance utilizing one or more newer characteristics. In this article, we will touch base upon the newer topical agents in the antifungal armamentarium and their unique properties which are different from the previous agents.

POLYENES

Lipid-based Amphotericin B Gel

Amphotericin B (AmB) has long been utilized for treatment of patients with invasive fungal infections but its severe toxicity restricted its use. Lipid-based delivery systems have made them safer for parenteral use.[1] Owing to the bulky

---

Email: ishanarang.d1@gmail.com

structure of AmB, its topical use is still limited due to lower transdermal absorption. AmB entrapped in charged liposomes has shown sustained skin absorption.[2] Lipid nanoparticles are designed to enhance drug delivery, chemical stability, and reduce the risk of toxicological problems and local irritancy.[3]

Sheikh et al. conducted a study to test a novel topical formulation of lipid-based AmB (0.1% AmB gel) was developed for safety, tolerability, and efficacy in adult patients with cutaneous and/or mucocutaneous fungal infection. On the basis of stability studies, they recommended shelf life of AmB gel is 24 months at 25°C. They assessed a total of 83 patients for cutaneous fungal infection where 39 patients were cured, 9 patients showed marked improvement, 26 patients showed moderate improvement, and 9 patients showed failure after the treatment. For mucocutaneous fungal infection, 100% patients were cured at the end of the treatment. No serious adverse events were reported in patients during the study.[4]

However, this is a study sponsored by a pharmaceutical industry and practically in the author's experience the result of the treatment is not promising.

AZOLE

Efinaconazole (Jublia)

Efinaconazole 10% solution is the Food and Drug Administration (FDA)-approved in the United States for the topical treatment of toenail onychomycosis caused by *Trichophyton rubrum* and *Trichophyton mentagrophytes* in June 2014.[5]

Since treatment of onychomycosis with efinaconazole may be for nearly a year, compliance and adherence to the treatment protocol are important for efficacy.[5] Table 1 briefly outlines various features of this drug.[5]

Eberconazole[6]

Eberconazole is an imidazole derivative, initially was launched in 2005 for the treatment of cutaneous mycoses (Table 2).

Eberconazole has broad spectrum of antifungal activity against yeast and fungi. Its anti-inflammatory action and efficacy against gram-positive bacteria can add to its efficacy in inflamed cutaneous mycoses and in secondary infections.

Luliconazole

Luliconazole 1% cream was approved in Japan in 2005 for the treatment of tinea and now in 2013 also approved by US FDA for the treatment of interdigital tinea pedis, tinea cruris, and tinea corporis caused by the organisms *T. rubrum* and *Epidermophyton floccosum*, in patients 18 years of age and older. In June 2009, the 1% cream was approved for marketing in India.[7]

Table 1: Salient Features of Efinaconazole[5]

Structure	• Member of the azole class (azoleamine derivative) • Molecular formula—$C_{18}H_{22}F_2N_{40}$
Human pharmacokinetics	• Slow absorption with lack of elimination phase • Metabolized to yield an H3 metabolite • Drug accumulates with successive applications and it usually takes five applications to reach steady state • Median half-life of efinaconazole and its metabolite at day 10 in healthy volunteers was 29.9 hours and 82.4 hours, respectively. Also, drug and its metabolite were detected in plasma 2 weeks after the final dose in patients with onychomycosis
Pharmacodynamics	• Cytochrome P450 enzyme inhibitor but clinically insignificant
Mechanism of action	• Inhibition of ergosterol synthesis via 14α-demethylase, with degenerative changes in hyphae secondarily
Spectrum of activity	• Dermatophytes, *Candida* species nondermatophyte molds
Potential use	• Mild-to-moderate DLSO onychomycosis
Efficacy	• Moderate antifungal activity but broader spectra than allylamines and morpholines • Antifungal activity against dermatophytes is comparable to terbinafine and amorolfine, higher activity against *Candida* species than itraconazole and has been comparable to terbinafine and more effective than amorolfine, ciclopirox, and itraconazole against nondermatophyte molds. 17-triazoles (such as fluconazole and itraconazole) had been used orally previously but not topically for the treatment of onychomycosis
Adverse effects	• Did not cause contact sensitization and induces only minimal skin irritation • High safety margin for topical treatment of onychomycosis
Safety	Pregnancy class C. It is excreted into breast milk, hence, FDA states that caution should be exercised in breastfeeding women

Table 2: Salient Features of Eberconazole[6]

Structure	• Broad-spectrum antifungal agent molecular formula $C_{18}H_{14}C_{12}N_2$
Human pharmacokinetics	• After topical application of eberconazole 2% cream in healthy
Mechanism of action	It inhibits ergosterol synthesis and has fungicidal or fungistatic activity depending on concentration. It is fungicidal at higher and fungistatic at lower concentrations
Spectrum of activity	• It has broad antimicrobial spectrum of activity against dermatophytes, *Candida* and *Malassezia furfur*. It has shown efficacy against most triazole resistant yeasts (*Candida krusei* and *Candida glabrata* and also fluconazole resistant *Candida albicans*. It is effective against gram-positive bacteria • It is distinct from other imidazoles as it has anti-inflammatory activity favoring use in inflamed dermatophytic infections
Efficacy	• Similar to clotrimazole, miconazole cream in treatment of dermatophytosis and candidiasis
Adverse effects	• Mild pruritus and burning sensation
Safety	• No significant systemic absorption

Luliconazole 1% cream once daily is effective even in short-term use (1 week for tinea corporis/cruris and 2 weeks for tinea pedis). A brief overview of the drug is mentioned in Table 3.[7]

The efficacy of luliconazole in dermatophyte infections appears to be equally good as with terbinafine and the other azoles and it will emerge as broad-spectrum antifungal in coming times.[7]

Table 3: Salient Features of Luliconazole[7]	
Structure	• Imidazole antifungal with unique structure • Imidazole moiety is incorporated in ketene dithioacetate structure
Human pharmacokinetics	• Optically related to lanoconazole • It is R-enantiomer which has more potent antifungal activity than racemic mixture of lanoconazole • It has good oral absorption, metabolic stability and low protein binding • Its therapeutic levels were achieved in an in vitro model *T. rubrum*-infected nail model within 7 days of daily dosing with 10% luliconazole solution • Low affinity for keratin and in contrast to many azoles, its potency remains unaffected by keratin
Mechanism of action	Inhibition of ergosterol synthesis via 14α-demethylase
Spectrum of activity	• Favorable antifungal activity against *Candida albicans*, *Malassezia* species, and *Aspergillus fumigatus* • Strong activity against *Trichophyton* species, similar to terbinafine
Potential use	Application of luliconazole 1% cream once daily is effective even in short-term use (1 week for tinea corporis/cruris and 2 weeks for tinea pedis)
Efficacy	• The MIC of luliconazole against *Trichophyton* species has been shown to be lower than most commonly used topical antifungals • The MIC of luliconazole against *Candida* species has been reported to be higher than that against filamentous fungi; however, it is similar to lanoconazole and greater than that of bifonazole, terbinafine and amorolfine • Similar to terbinafine, luliconazole has strong fungicidal activity against *Trichophyton* species. Its strong clinical antifungal activity of luliconazole is possibly attributable to a combination of strong in vitro antifungal activity and favorable pharmacokinetic properties in the skin
Adverse effects	• Excellent local tolerability and a lack of systemic side effects with topical use
Safety	• Favorable safety profile • Occasional mild application site reactions

Sertaconazole[8]

Sertaconazole is also an imidazole antifungal agent with both fungistatic and fungicidal activity depending on the concentration. Sertaconazole 2% cream was approved by the FDA in 2003 for the treatment of tinea pedis in individuals aged 12 years or more. It has similar spectrum of activity like the other azoles. Its recommended usage is 2% sertaconazole cream applied once or twice daily for 4 weeks.

Pramiconazole[8]

Pramiconazole is a newer triazole under development with activity against dermatophytes, *Candida* and *Malassezia*. Both oral and topical preparations of pramiconazole have shown promising efficacy compared to itraconazole and terbinafine against *Microsporum canis* in animal studies.[8]

OXABOROLES

Tavaborole (Kerydin)[9]

Tavaborole was approved by the US FDA in July 2014 for topical treatment of mild-to-moderate toenail onychomycosis daily for 48 weeks (Table 4).

UPCOMING DRUGS AND FORMULATIONS

Newer investigational drugs are mentioned in Table 5.

Table 4: Salient Features of Tavaborole[9]	
Structure	Boron containing structure; 5-fluoro-1,3-dihydro-1-hydroxy-2,1-benzoxaborole
Human pharmacokinetics	It has smaller molecular weight and so a greater nail plate penetration than its predecessor
Pharmacodynamics	Did not inhibit the cytochrome P450 isoforms
Mechanism of action	Interferes with fungal protein synthesis by interfering with cytoplasmic leucyl-transfer RNA synthetase
Spectrum of activity	Dermatophytes—*T. mentagrophytes* and *T. rubrum, T. tonsurans, Epidermophyton floccosum, M. audouinii, M. canis* and *M. gypseum* (2 µg/mL). 41 nondermatophytic molds, such as *Aspergillus fumigatus* and *Fusarium solani*, and yeast such as *Candida albicans*
Potential use	• Licensed for mild-to-moderate toenail onychomycosis • Although its mycologic cure rate is lower than oral antifungal agents it offers an adjuncts as well as an alternative to available topical antifungal therapies
Efficacy	Head-to-head comparison studies are required in future
Adverse effects	Application site exfoliation, application site erythema and dermatitis
Safety	Excellent safety profile

Table 5: Investigational Antifungal Drugs[8]						
Drug	Mechanism of action	Concentration and vehicle	Phase of clinical trial	Indications	Results of clinical trials	Spectrum of antimicrobial activity other than antidermatophytic
Arasertacon-azole	14α-lanosterol demethylase inhibitor	–	Animal model	–	Very potent in vitro activity against dermatophytes	• Vulvovaginal candidiasis • Antifungal • Antibacterial
BB2603	Squalene epoxidase inhibition	Spray	Phase I/II	Onychomycosis and associated tinea pedis	Ongoing	–
ME1111	Succinate dehydrogenase inhibition	0.06–32 mg/L	In vitro	–	Significant anti-dermatophytic action	–
AR12 (OSU-03012)	Acetyl-CoA synthetase inhibitor	5% (w/v)	Phase I	Onychomycosis	–	• Antifungal activity (Candida species, Cryptococcus, Blastomyces, Histoplasma and Coccidioides) • Antibacterial (Salmonella and Francisella) • Antiparasitic (Leishmania donovani) • Antiviral

Continued

Continued

Table 5: Investigational Antifungal Drugs[8]

SB208	Cell death stimulants; Nitric oxide donors	2%, 4%, 12% gel once daily for 2 weeks	Phase II	Interdigital tinea pedis	Statistically significant effect compared to vehicle	–
CD101 (Echinocandins)	Glucan synthase inhibitors	Subcutaneous, 10–40 mg/kg/week, 2 doses	Animal model	Inoculum put over abraded area over back	Significant clinical and mycological efficacy compared to the vehicle	Systemic candidemia
NB-002	Mechanically destabilize fungal hyphae	0.25%, and 0.5% emulsion	Phase II	Distal subungual onychomycosis	Completed, no results available	*Candida albicans Paecilomyces lilacinus, Fusarium* species, *Scedosporium* species, and *Scopulariopsis* species
Hydroxychavicol	Disruption of cell membrane integrity	–	In vitro	–	Significant anti-dermatophytic action	*Candida parapsilosis*
Phlorotannins	• Affect ergosterol composition of cell membrane • Affect the respiratory chain function	–	In vitro	–	Significant anti-dermatophytic action	*Candida* species

Source: Sahni K, Singh S, Dogra S. Newer topical treatments in skin and nail dermatophyte infections. *Indian Dermatol Online J.* 2018;9(3):149-58.

CONCLUSION

Apart from the newer agents in older classes of antifungal drugs like azoles, polyenes, etc. we also have developed newer classes of antifungals like oxaboroles. In future, we expect more newer classes of antifungals. But at some point we do recognize that the older antifungals will still remain the go-to agents.

REFERENCES

1. Azanza J, Sadada B, Reis J. Liposomal formulations of amphotericin B: differences according to the scientific evidence. *Rev Esp Quimioter.* 2015;28(6):275-281.
2. Manosroi A, Kongkaneramit L, Manosroi J. Stability and transdermal absorption of topical amphotericin B liposome formulations. *Int J Pharm.* 2004;270(1-2):279-286.
3. Muller RH, Radtke M, Wissing SA. Solid lipid nanoparticles (SLN) and nanostructured lipid carriers (NLC) in cosmetic and dermatological preparations. *Adv Drug Deliv Rev.* 2002;54 Suppl 1:S131-155.
4. Sheikh S, Ahmad A, Ali S, Paithankar M, Raval R. Topical Delivery of Lipid Based Amphotericin B Gel in the Treatment of Fungal Infection: A Clinical Efficacy, Safety and Tolerability Study in Patients. *J Clin Exp Dermatol Res.* 2014(5):248.
5. Lipner SR, Scher RK. Efinaconazole in the treatment of onychomycosis. *Infection and drug resistance.* 2015;8:163-172.
6. Moodahadu-Bangera LS, Martis J, Mittal R, et al. Eberconazole--pharmacological and clinical review. Indian *journal of dermatology, venereology and leprology.* 2012;78(2):217-222.
7. Khanna D, Bharti S. Luliconazole for the treatment of fungal infections: an evidence-based review. *Core Evid.* 2014;9:113-124.
8. Sahni K, Singh S, Dogra S. Newer topical treatments in skin and nail dermatophyte infections. *Indian Dermatol Online J.* 2018;9(3):149-158.
9. Jinna S, Finch J. Spotlight on tavaborole for the treatment of onychomycosis. *Drug Des Devel Ther.* 2015;9:6185-6190.

World Clin Dermatol. 2019;5(1):135-40.

Counseling for Dermatophytosis: Is it Important in Today's Scenario?

[1],*Neha Dubey MD, [2]Akansha Bhargava MD

[1]Consultant Dermatologist, Medanta The Medicity Hospital and Meraki Skin Clinic, Gurugram, Haryana, India
[2]Department of Dermatology, Venereology and Leprosy, Bundelkhand Medical College, Sagar, Madhya Pradesh, India

ABSTRACT

The ever-changing clinical scenario of dermatophytosis poses a constant threat of treatment failure, resistance and recurrence. Although patient counseling forms an integral part of treatment of any disease, be it dermatological or nondermatological, this art seems to succumb to the lack of time both on the doctor's as well as patient's part. This article explains why and how a patient seeking treatment of dermatophytosis can benefit from a good counseling by the dermatologist at the time of commencement of treatment.

INTRODUCTION

Dermatophytosis is a fungal infection, affecting keratinized tissues such as superficial layer of epidermis, hair and nail. The recent prevalence rate of dermatophytosis in India ranges from 36.6% to 78.4%.[1] With the current alarming situation of enormous increase in the incidence as well as the prevalence of superficial dermatophytosis over the past 4–5 years across the country, it is safe to regard it as more of a public health problem. Various studies done on dermatophytosis in different cities in India suggest the same.[2-5] The clinical pattern of dermatophytosis has undergone a sea change in the hands of unstable environmental factors, increased prevalence of *Trichophyton mentagrophytes*

*Corresponding author
Email: nehadubey1101@gmail.com

causing more inflamed lesions and resistance to antifungal agents.[6,7] Adding to this situation, irrational use of fixed drug combination creams containing antifungal, steroid (often a potent one like Clobetasol propionate) and an antibacterial is making things more difficult.[7-11] All this makes counseling of a patient suffering from dermatophytosis very important in today's time (Table 1).

Table 1: Measures to be Explained while Counseling a Patient of Dermatophytosis[13,22-24]	
Measures	**Reason**
Avoiding topical antifungal preparations with steroid combinations	Causes decreased local immunologic host reaction which may lead to persistence of infection and deeper invasion of tissue
Stress should be given on the importance of regularity of medication and adherence to the advice of the physician	For better compliance
Topical antifungals should be applied 2 cm beyond the margins of tinea for 2 weeks beyond clinical resolution	To prevent recurrence
Strictly avoiding tight garments such as jeans, leggings and jeggings. Encourage patient to wear loose cotton garments	To avoid moisture because of perspiration
Discourage sharing bed linens, towels and clothes	To avoid spread of infection from patient to another person and vice versa
Use of hot water for washing clothes and bed linen and drying them in sun. Ironing can be opted in case of absence of sunlight. Infected clothes should be washed separately	Most dermatophytes grow poorly at 37°C
Instruct patient of tinea cruris to wear boxer shorts instead of tight fitted ones and occlusive footwear to be avoided in cases of tinea pedis	To avoid moisture due to perspiration
Use of absorbent powders and deodorants in cases of tinea cruris	It decreases perspiration
Proper vacuuming, dusting and wet mopping of the house	It reduces the spore load in the environment
Careful history to be taken to rule out similar complaints in family members	Treatment of family members is important to avoid reinfection
Regularly trim nails and minimize trauma and avoid sharing nail clippers	For better penetration of antifungal nail lacquer and to avoid spread of infection

Note: Distribution of pamphlets and posters to patients can ensure strict adherence to all the above mentioned measures.

FACTORS THAT MAKE PATIENT COUNSELING THE NEED OF THE HOUR

Changing Clinical Pattern

Steroid-modified tinea in India is turning out to be more of an epidemic. The usual pattern followed by most of the patients is going to the nearby pharmacist upon first noticing the infection, looking for an easily available over the counter preparation which would provide quick relief. The pharmacist, in turn, on most occasions suggests a combination of topical antifungal with antibacterial and a potent steroid.[6,7]

These steroid formulations suppress the cutaneous inflammatory response mounted by the skin while fighting the dermatophyte. Parallelly, the T-cell mediated immune response to the dermatophyte is also suppressed, therefore, leading to the altered clinical patterns of dermatophytosis which are widespread, chronic and inadequately eliminated which we have been witnessing over the last few years (Table 2).

All of this makes patient education and counseling regarding steroid abuse and avoiding over the counter products a priority.

Changing Pattern of Dermatophytes

The face of dermatophytosis in India has transformed over the recent years. *Trichophyton mentagrophytes* have been identified as the predominant causative organism in various mycological studies undertaken across the country lately.[14-18] Some studies have also changed our perspective of the role of fomites in transmission of dermatophytosis. A study showed, *T. rubrum* surviving for less than 12 weeks on a towel while *T. mentagrophytes* survived for greater than 25 weeks.[19] This highlights the indispensable role counseling can play in proper patient care, thus, informing the patient about the importance of disinfection of clothes, best done by washing them in hot water and drying them in sunlight, as it is the most effective disinfectant for dermatophytes.[20]

Table 2: Factors Responsible for Propagation of Dermatophytosis[12,13]
• Geographic location and habits: Hot and humid climate, use of occlusive wear
• Genetic predisposition
• Immunosuppression
• Virulence of organism

Prevailing Fashion Trends

The ongoing fashion promotes the use of tight fitting clothing such as jeggings, leggings and denims by youngsters who generally are not so concerned about the practical aspects like their incompatibility to hot and humid climate. This seems to be the most relevant explanation to the increased prevalence of tinea corporis and tinea cruris not only in the overweight individuals but also in otherwise fit and otherwise hygiene conscious patients with no other risk factors (Table 3).

Hence, it makes a lot of sense to counsel the patient about the suitable clothing material that can add to the efficacy of the treatment.

Increased Spore Load within Families

It is noteworthy that while in the past, tinea capitis was considered to be the most common fungal infection occurring in children,[13] these days it is not startling to see large sized lesions and multiple site involvement in them. This has happened because the spore load within the families has increased considering multiple family members being affected at the same time. This also confirms the role of fomites, especially in case of pediatric patients in whom sharing of linens and clothing is common. We also can't ignore the fact that the virulence of the organism has also increased. Therefore, it is of utmost importance to elicit a careful family history in all patients as an undocumented and untreated affected family member can be a source of constant reinfection.

WHY COUNSELING IS BENEFICIAL TO THE PATIENT?

The transformation of dermatophytosis in India is an outcome of a complex interplay between the host, fungus, environment and to a major extent drugs also. To top it all, even the agricultural industry uses antifungals on a widescale, and the role of antifungal drug resistance cannot be denied.[8,21,22] As a result of all this and due to sheer ignorance on the patient's part the lesions may become widespread and may create negative social and psychological effects, thus significantly effecting the quality of life. All this can be avoided by counseling the patient on every visit

Table 3: A Proper Counseling Result
• Better patient understanding of their disease and the role of medication in treatment
• Improved medical adherence
• More effective drug treatment
• Reduced incidence of adverse effects and unnecessary healthcare costs

and providing them the required information about the nature of their disease and how they can also contribute to their fast recovery by changing some of their habits and following few instructions.

Challenges

Because of rapid emergence of rare dermatophyte species which mimic other clinical diseases, their evaluation is critical to establish the diagnosis.[25]

The increase in numbers of individuals with low immunity and people with more susceptibility for fungal infections, there is a pressure being generated on the cost of health care.

Availability of cheaper over the counter formulations (steroid-containing) provides quick relief but making the disease worse and resistant to standard anti-fungals.

Prescribing topical and oral antifungals in suboptimum and irrational regimens by general practitioners.

CONCLUSION

Communication often holds the missing link to success and should not be overlooked.[26] In today's practice, the burden of difficulty to treat dermatophytosis is increasing, so it is important to stress upon patient's counseling along with oral and topical antifungal agents, which will benefit both the patient as well as the treating dermatologist.

REFERENCES

1. Naglot A, Shrimali DD, Nath BK, et al. Recent trends of Dermatophytosis in Northeast India (Assam) and interpretation with published studies. *Int J Curr Microbiol App Sci.* 2015;4:111-20.
2. Das K, Basak S, Ray S. A study on superficial fungal infection from West Bengal: A brief report. *J Life Sci.* 2009;1:51-5.
3. Nawal P, Patel S, Patel M, Soni S, Khandelwal N. A study of superficial mycosis in tertiary care hospital. *Natl J Integr Res Med.* 2012;3:95-9.
4. Chudasama V, Solanki H, Vadasmiya M, Javadekar T. A study of superficial mycosis in tertiary care hospital. *Int J Sci Res.* 2014;3:222-4.
5. Narasimhalu CR, Kalyani M, Somendar S. A cross-sectional, clinico-mycological research study of prevalence, aetiology, speciation and sensitivity of superficial fungal infection in Indian patients. *J Clin Exp Dermatol Res.* 2016;7:324.
6. Verma SB. Sales, status, prescriptions and regulatory problems with topical steroids in India. *Indian J Dermatol Venereol Leprol.* 2014;80:201-3.
7. Verma SB. Topical steroid misuse in India is harmful and out of control. *BMJ.* 2015;351:h6079.
8. Dogra S, Uprety S. The menace of chronic and recurrent dermatophytosis in India: Is the problem deeper than we perceive? *Indian Dermatol Online J.* 2016;7:73-6.

9. Lahiri K, Coondoo A. Topical and steroid damaged/dependent face(TSDF): An entity of cutaneous pharmacodependence. *Indian J Dermatol.* 2016;61:265-72.

10. Rathi SK, D'Souza P. Rational and ethical use of topical corticosteroids based on safety and efficacy. *Indian J Dermatol.* 2012;57:251-9.

11. Kumar S, Goyal A, Gupta YK. Abuse of topical corticosteroids in India: Concerns and the way forward. *J Pharmacol Pharmacother.* 2016;7:7-15.

12. Hay RJ, Roberts SoB, Mackenzie DWR. Mycology. In: Champion RH, Burton JL, Ebling FJG, editors. Textbook of dermatology. Oxford: Blackwell Scientific Publication; 1992. pp.1128.

13. Manjunath Shenoy M, Suchitra Shenoy M. Superficial fungal infections. In: Sacchidanand S, Oberoi C, Inamdar AC, editors. IADVL Textbook of Dermatology. 4th edition. Mumbai: Bhalani Publishing House; 2015. pp. 459-516.

14. Kansra S. Prevalence of dermatophytosis and their antifungal susceptibility in a tertiary care hospital of North India. *Int J Sci Res.* 2016;5:450-3

15. Khan MS, Khan N. A study of fungal isolates from superficial mycoses cases attending IIMS & R, Lucknow. *Int J Life Sci Sci Res.* 2016;2:37-42.

16. Agarwal US, Saran J, Agarwal P. Clinico-mycological study of dermatophytes in a tertiary care centre in Northwest India. *Indian J Dermatol Venereol Leprol.* 2014;80:194.

17. Kaur I, Thakur K, Sood A, et al. Clinico-mycological profile of clinically diagnosed cases of dermatophytosis in North India: A prospective cross-sectional study. *Int J Health Sci Res.* 2016;6:54-60.

18. Noronha TM, Tophakhane RS, Nadiger S. Clinico-microbiological study of dermatophytosis in a tertiary-care hospital in North Karnataka. *Indian Dermatol Online J.* 2016;7:264-7.

19. Khanjanasthiti P, Srisawat P. Germination and survival of dermatophyte spores in various environmental conditions. *Chiang Mai Med.* 1984;23:83-98

20. Amichai B, Grunwald MH, Davidovici B, Shemer A. Sunlight is said to be the best of disinfectants: The efficacy of sun exposure for reducing fungal contamination in used clothes. *Isr Med Assoc J.* 2014;16:431-3.

21. Verma S, Madhu R. The great Indian epidemic of superficial dermatophytosis: an appraisal. *Indian J Dermatol.* 2017;62:227–36

22. Zhan P, Liu W. The changing face of Dermatophytic infections worldwide. *Mycopathologia.* 2017;182:77-86.

23. Ameen M, Lear JT, Madan V, Mohd Mustapa MF, Richardson M. British Association of Dermatologists guidelines for the management of onychomycosis 2014. *Br J Dermatol.* 2014;937-58.

24. Gupta AK, Foley KA, Versteeg SG. New Antifungal Agents and new Formulations Against Dermatophytes. *Mycopathologia.* 2017;182:127-41.

25. Bhagra S, Ganju SA, Kanga A, Sharma NL, Guleria RC. Mycological pattern of dermatophytosis in and around Shimla hills. *Indian J Dermatol.* 2014;59:268-70.

26. OhioLINK. (2003). An exploration of the pharmacist-patient communicative relationship. [online]. Available from https://etd.ohiolink.edu/ap/10?0::NO:10:P10_ACCESSION_NUM:osu1061259087 [Last accessed February 2019]

WORLD CLINICS
Statement of Purpose

The streams of medicine and surgery are evolving constantly at a rapid pace, creating a need for the healthcare professionals to continuously update their knowledge base and skills. This is necessary to offer their patients the best 'real world' treatment options based on current concepts, status, and trends, reflecting the achievements of evidence-based medicine. This pace of advances in medicine is a compelling reason for the physicians and surgeons to seek information through multiple resources such as journals, workshops and conferences.

WORLD CLINICS are periodicals of evidence-based reviews proposed as a source of comprehensive, state-of-the art reviews written by experts representing the global academia under the mentorship of an Editor-in-Chief. The comments by the 'Guest Editor' (or Editor-in-Chief) given at the end of each article/chapter would be representative of their clinical experience. Each issue of "WORLD CLINICS Dermatology" would focus on a single theme covering topics that are relevant to clinical understanding and decision-making. Each topic would be developed to reflect the current evidence, research, existing guidelines and recommendations as well the clinical experience of experts.

Objectives

- Provide up-to-date reviews on disease management, technique, procedure, or technology.
- Help enhance knowledge and skill for application in clinical practice.
- To aid use of evidence in decision-making for improved patient care.
- To help select best treatment options and overcome treatment challenges.

Target Readers

WORLD CLINICS are meant for practicing physicians, fellows, and postgraduate students, who plan to keep abreast with the current best-evidence clinical practices that are recommended and followed by experts globally.

Periodicity

WORLD CLINICS Dermatology will be released with a frequency of two issues per year.

Themes

Each subject area of WORLD CLINICS will cover themes on any of the following:

1. A disease or a disorder (e.g., Acne) OR
2. An organ or an anatomical region (e.g., Wrist, in WORLD CLINICS Orthopedics) OR
3. A technique or a treatment approach (e.g., Various methods for the treatment of CTEV, in WORLD CLINICS Orthopedics) OR
4. A special population group (e.g., Management of HIV infected pregnant patients in WORLD CLINICS Obstetrics and Gynecology) OR
5. A technology (e.g., 3D Ultrasound in diagnosis of gynecological abnormalities in WORLD CLINICS Obstetrics and Gynecology)

WORLD CLINICS
Manuscript Guidelines for Authors

General Guidelines

- Manuscripts must be typed in double-space including all text, references, tables, and figure legends, and should be sent in a single word file.
- For any copyright work, the necessary permissions must be obtained by the author and sent along with the manuscript. These permissions apply to any borrowed, modified, or adapted text, tables, or figures.
- For any production-quality artwork (images, illustrations, etc.) please see the guidelines under images.
- Acknowledgments or disclosures, if required, should be cited before the references.

Author Credits

- Should be in the first page.
- Each author's name, degree, academic or professional affiliation, city, and state (or country).
- E-mail address, mailing address, and telephone number of each co-author.
- If more than one author, mention the corresponding author.
- Please supply 4–6 keywords which will be used to optimize search results.

Subheads

The format for article's headings and subheadings is as follows:
'A' head: All caps, bold.
'B' head: Title case (upper/lower), bold.
'C' head: Title case (upper/lower), bold, italics.
'D' head: Title case (upper lower), normal, Roman.
'E' head: Sentence case (initial letter capital), italics, run in.

References

- References must be cited sequentially only at the end of the manuscript in the order as they appear in the text.
- Follow the Vancouver style for the references, using the Index Medicus abbreviations for journals that are indexed; if a journal is not indexed, use full name.
- If there are more than six authors, cite first six and add "et al."

    e.g., Lacasse Y, Selman M, Costabel U, Dalphin JC, Ando M, Morell F, et al. Clinical Diagnosis of Hypersensitivity Pneumonitis. *Am J Respir Crit Care Med*. 2003;168:952-8.

Images

- There is generally no restriction on number of boxes, tables, or images, but keep them to a minimum necessary.
- A maximum of two hand-drawn illustrations and maximum of two algorithms are allowed.
- Medium for delivery of photographs: Individual TIFF or JPEG files each at a resolution no lower than 300 dpi (118 pixels/cm) when viewed at 100 mm width.
- The images and illustrations can also be in full color.